THE FACTS ABOUT HYSTERECTOMY

Did you know:

• Hysterectomy is second only to caesarean section in surgical procedures most commonly practiced in the United States.

• Many hysterectomies are being performed unnecessarily, and having the facts is your best assurance that the treatment you receive is right for you.

• At current rates, one out of every three women can expect to have a hysterectomy before reaching age 65.

The best medicine begins with informed consumers. If you or someone you love is facing surgery, give the gift of information—the key to good health.

THE WELL-INFORMED PATIENT'S GUIDE TO HYSTERECTOMY

THE DELL SURGICAL LIBRARY:

THE WELL-INFORMED PATIENT'S GUIDE TO HYSTERECTOMY

THE WELL-INFORMED PATIENT'S GUIDE TO CORONARY BYPASS SURGERY

THE WELL-INFORMED PATIENT'S GUIDE TO BUNION AND OTHER FOOT SURGERY

THE WELL-INFORMED PATIENT'S GUIDE TO CAESAREAN BIRTHS

THE WELL-INFORMED PATIENT'S GUIDE TO CATARACT AND OTHER EYE SURGERY

THE WELL-INFORMED PATIENT'S GUIDE TO SURGERY FOR KNEE AND OTHER SPORTS INJURIES

DELL SURGICAL LIBRARY

THE WELL-INFORMED PATIENT'S GUIDE TO

HYSTERECTOMY

KATHRYN COX, M.D., AND JUDITH D. SCHWARTZ

A DELL BOOK

Published by
Dell Publishing
a division of
Bantam Doubleday Dell Publishing Group, Inc.
666 Fifth Avenue
New York, New York 10103

This book is not intended as a substitute for medical advice of physicians and should be used only in conjunction with the advice of your
personal doctor. The reader should regularly consult a physician in
matters relating to his or her health and particularly with respect to
any symptoms that may require diagnosis or medical attention.

Published by arrangement with G. S. Sharpe Communications, Inc.,
606 West 116 Street, New York, New York 10027

ISBN: 0-440-20715-0

Printed in the United States of America

Published simultaneously in Canada

April 1991

10 9 8 7 6 5 4 3 2

OPM

Contents

Introduction

Today the mere mention of the word *hysterectomy* is bound to provoke a heated response. In the last few years, a number of reports have come out both in the popular press and in the medical literature charging that a sizable percentage of hysterectomies performed cannot be medically justified. Considering that the number of hysterectomies hovers around 650,000 annually— making it the second most common surgical procedure in the United States, behind caesarean sections—an alarming number of women may be operated on with no apparent benefit to their health, and sometimes, as we shall see, to the detriment of it.

A woman who is told by her gynecologist that a hysterectomy is in order may well feel caught in the middle of this conflict: she has heard horrible stories about women who lose their hopes of having children, lose their bladder function, lose their sex lives—all for an operation of dubious intent. She may begin to question her doctor, which can in itself be disconcerting since, after all, this is the person in whom she's entrusted her health. She is concerned about her physical well-being, about her fibroids, endometriosis, risk of cancer, or whatever has led her doctor to recommend surgery in the first place. In short, she's frightened about the consequences of having the operation—and of not having it. And the result is often confusion, or anger.

The point for every woman to bear in mind is that while hysterectomy raises many political issues—women's rights or how the medical establishment treats women—it is primarily a medical issue. In many instances the surgical removal of the uterus *is* the best option for a woman's health. Not even the harshest critic of hysterectomies can deny that the operation has saved countless women undue pain, and for many it has indeed saved their lives.

Hysterectomy is also overwhelmingly a personal issue. In all but perhaps 15 percent of cases, generally when cancer is present or suspected, having or not having a hysterectomy is not a life-or-death situation. What is at stake, rather, is quality of life. A number of factors must be weighed in the decision about surgery, among them the woman's age, her wish to have children, her level of present discomfort, the level of risk for serious illnesses, and last, but in no way least, how she *feels* about having her uterus and possibly ovaries removed. It's usually a matter of balancing risk and alternatives, comfort and a desire to save her organs. In some instances, given two women with similar medical diagnoses, one may be a good candidate for a hysterectomy while the other may prove not to be.

Today the *rate* of hysterectomies seems to be dipping slightly. (The *number* is staying about the same, since the number of women in the age-group with the highest hysterectomy rate—those aged forty to forty-five—is rising as baby boomers hit their forties.)

One reason for this is that medical science is offering more alternatives. Procedures that were mere technological visions a decade ago (various applications of lasers, for instance) can sometimes save women the pain and risk of major invasive surgery. Operations that were all but neglected in most cases (such as a myomectomy, which removes fibroid tumors while leaving the uterus intact) have made their way into the medical mainstream, giving many women the option of retaining their reproductive organs and maintaining their fertility.

With the frequency of hysterectomies being called into question, the medical community has had to retrain its thinking. Increasingly, physicians are encouraged to explore alternatives and then determine which approach will suit the woman in question—and not simply yank out body parts at the first hint of illness. This orientation stresses the woman's health, not only her potential for disease.

The key to the recent decline in hysterectomies is that women have made an effort to learn more about their bodies. We've become active medical consumers, so that we question our doctors' opinions rather than submit passively to surgery. Women's groups have worked to inform us and to initiate legislation that would protect women from unnecessary dangers. For example, in 1987, California passed a law requiring women to grant oral and written consent before having a hysterectomy. In some cases women have won lawsuits from physicians who failed to warn them of potential side effects of surgery. Thirty years ago if a woman was found to have fibroids, her gynecologist might, without hesitation, have insisted that the uterus be removed. That's less likely to happen today.

But there's a long way to go. There are still doctors who are cavalier toward women and insensitive about their patients' bodies. There are areas of the country where a woman is far more likely to undergo a hysterectomy. Many experts suggest that a particularly high regional rate may reflect unnecessary surgery. (The operation is most common in the South, least common in the Northeast.) Despite ample documentation in the medical literature, there is still a debate about whether many of the reported side effects—waning interest in sex, depression, fatigue—are medically derived or whether they're "all in the patient's head." And, not surprisingly, a great deal of confusion among women persists.

At current rates, one out of every three women can expect to have a hysterectomy before reaching age sixty-five. Many more will at some point in their lives be confronted with the decision. A hysterectomy is *not* minor surgery, and no woman should be forced into having one without fully appreciating what's involved—psychologically as well as physiologically. All this makes it especially important that a woman work *with* her doctor to determine the best course of action. Women who take part in the decision to undergo surgery tend to suffer fewer emotional side effects than those who feel steamrolled into it. The sense of personal loss arising from the removal of internal organs appears to be heightened when there's a sense that they've been taken—even stolen—away. Only by taking control of your own health can you insure that what you do will be the best thing for you, and that you'll be comfortable with the outcome.

In this book, we aim to clear away some of the confusion surrounding hysterectomies. We hope to answer most of your questions about the procedure, alternative treatments, and aftereffects, both short- and long-term. This book is neither a defense of hysterectomies nor a political treatise against them. Rather we wish to provide clear, straightforward guidance to help you come to an informed, confident decision concerning the place of hysterectomy in your life.

The book is intended for anyone facing the possibility of hysterectomy, anyone close to a woman who is a candidate for hysterectomy, or anyone who has had one and still wishes to know more. We've written it to be both comprehensive and clear, and sufficiently readable to be gone through cover to cover. In general, we recommend that you read the entire book because so many issues are of interest to all women considering hysterectomy. If you're looking for more specific information, however, you can turn straight to the chapter concerned.

Number of hysterectomies

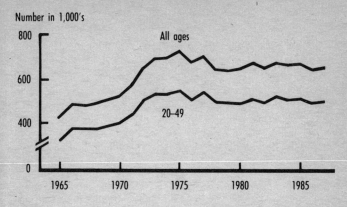

Number in 1,000's

All ages

20–49

SOURCE: NCHS, National Hospital Discharge Survey, 1965–87

Rate of hysterectomies by age

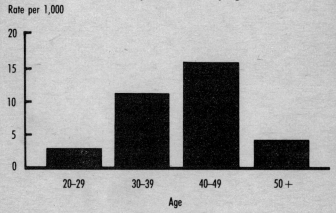

Rate per 1,000

Age

SOURCE: NCHS, National Hospital Discharge Survey, 1985–87

CHAPTER 1

Hysterectomy: The Controversy in Context

A little over a year ago, Patricia, forty, went to her physician complaining of pelvic pain. Upon finding a dermoid cyst on the ovary, a benign condition, the doctor recommended a hysterectomy. "You don't want any more children," he reminded her. "So why leave the uterus in when it's only going to cause problems?" This was a bit more drastic a measure than she had had in mind, and she was somewhat taken aback by his response.

Because her insurance company required a second opinion before covering surgery, she saw another doctor. This one carefully spelled out the pros and cons of a hysterectomy for her condition, explaining that in such cases it's often an individual decision whether or not to do anything other than remove the ovary. Many

women with benign ovarian conditions choose a hyster-
ectomy if they have other problems, such as bleeding or
fibroids, and are more comfortable with the uterus
removed. The initial doctor wasn't necessarily wrong,
he explained, he just wasn't giving her the complete
picture—with the full spectrum of alternatives.

Just having this clarified put Patricia at ease. Before,
she had felt there was something wrong with her; now
she felt she understood what she was facing and what
her options were.

Maura, thirty-eight, had been fighting what seemed
to be a never-ending battle against endometriosis. At age
twenty-two and then at age thirty-two, she had surgery to
remove the adhesions. On top of that, she was put on birth
control pills and Danocrine. The medication gave her
uncomfortable side effects, but without it she was in
constant pain. In short, she was at the end of her rope.

Single and with no plans for a family, she and her
doctor decided that a hysterectomy might be the an-
swer. After the operation she felt great—freed for the
first time from symptoms that had long plagued her.
But a few months later she read an article about unnec-
essary hysterectomies, and suddenly she started won-
dering whether she had made a mistake, whether she
was just another statistic.

One reason hysterectomies are so controversial today
is that for a long time doctors were treating women
patients as though the loss of their uterus and/or ovaries

was a matter of no significance. When uncomfortable physical or emotional side effects arose—as they do nearly 50 percent of the time—doctors often dismissed them as a lack of adjustment or emotional stability on the part of the woman; indeed, as though it were her fault. In the doctors' view, the uterus, the source of the "problem," was removed, so the woman should be thankful and no longer suffer. Because of a common tendency in medicine to use surgery aggressively, the prevailing view has been "when in doubt, take it out." In this way many doctors were inclined to treat merely the *anatomical* woman and not the *whole* woman, which includes her emotional self as well as her physical self.

But on many levels, losing one's uterus and/or ovaries is far more devastating than losing any other organ that can be lived without, such as tonsils or an appendix; studies reveal that women have had much greater difficulty adjusting from a hysterectomy than, for example, from a gall bladder operation. For one thing, the uterus is an integral part of a woman's female identity and, regardless of age, a post-hysterectomy patient may feel "less of a woman" without it. (It's worth noting that, technically, the removal of ovaries in a woman is equivalent to a man's losing his testicles—in other words, to castration. Is it likely that a male doctor would be so nonchalant about a male patient's undergoing such an operation?)

About 60 percent of women who have hysterectomies are under the age of forty-five. Without her uterus, a woman cannot conceive and give birth. After a hysterectomy, women of childbearing age frequently face a period of depression or mourning. Some physicians have figured that once a woman has had as many children as she wants, the loss of her uterus should not cause any emotional trauma. But the emotional response may have little to do with the *reality* of having more children and may instead be tied to the possibility or even the fantasy of having children. And having these taken away abruptly and prematurely may be tremendously upsetting.

Also, for some women the uterus and/or the cervix—the tip of the uterus that extends to the upper part of the vagina—plays a role in their experience of sex. While many women derive most of their pleasurable sensations during sex from the stimulation of the clitoris, for others pleasure is centered on the movements and rhythmic contractions of the uterus or stimulation of the cervix. Studies and reports from women make it clear that hysterectomy does have an effect on sex. For many women the effect is a positive one, often the result of being freed from pelvic pain or from the bother of contraception. But to claim that sex *doesn't* or *shouldn't* be altered by a hysterectomy—as many physicians and so-called experts have—is not facing the facts. Women who undergo the operation need to be made aware that there's a possibility that their sex lives could be affected.

Then there are physiological changes, many of which are not fully understood. Once her ovaries are taken out (as they are in 25 percent of all women with hysterectomies, more than 50 percent among those over forty), a woman in her childbearing years confronts a sudden, surgically induced menopause, and all the physical and emotional changes that go with it. Many symptoms associated with menopause (although by no means do all women experience them), such as headaches, depression, and hot flashes, hit younger women especially hard because hormone levels plummet so rapidly.

But even if a woman has been through menopause, her ovaries still produce hormones, albeit in smaller quantities. And in terms of hormone secretion the function of the uterus is not yet clear, although recent studies suggest it may play a role or may in some way contribute to ovarian hormone production. What *does* seem clear is that at no time are the uterus and ovaries inert, easily expendable organs. Many physicians maintain that estrogen replacement therapy (ERT) will take care of any hormonal disruptions. But in no way can this be viewed as a panacea. For one thing, the balance of hormones in the body is quite complex, with much yet to be learned. And although usually well tolerated, estrogen therapy is not without risks (see Chapter 12, The Question of Hormone Therapy).

Besides all of the unknowns, what *is* known is that a hysterectomy is a major operation, and like any operation involving surgery and anesthesia it entails some risk of complications and mortality. About one in a thousand patients undergoing a hysterectomy will die as a result of surgery. True, this is a more favorable rate than that for many operations, but depending on the medical need for it in a given situation, surgery may represent a greater hazard than would a more conservative approach. Also, the rate of complications following hysterectomy is fairly high. Minor infections, principally bladder infections, and fever soon after surgery are not uncommon, and damage to other pelvic organs can, though rarely, occur. But how many women are fully informed of such risks before offering their bodies up to surgery?

In light of these risks and realities, it might seem absurd that physicians have been so ready to reach for the knife. The possible explanation for this is complex, reflecting both a long-standing attitude on the part of doctors toward women and various tendencies and pressures within the medical community. The controversy started as women over the last few decades began reacting to what they perceived as a needless assault on their bodies. And it continues to brew as the medical establishment shows a willingness to question and address its own excesses. All these changes should prove very positive for women.

But, for the individual dealing with her own health and her own future, today's climate of controversy can be unsettling. With views from her doctors, her friends, and the media coming at her from all directions, whom is she to believe? Who really knows what's best for her, and who can supply the information she needs?

The two examples at the beginning of this chapter clearly demonstrate this state of puzzlement. Patricia truly wanted to take her doctor's word. He had delivered both of her babies and had always been conscientious in treating her. But she felt disturbed, even betrayed, when he appeared to be callous about advising a hysterectomy, in her view acting as if the uterus were nothing more than a torn garment to be tossed out. It's important to note that doctors who entered the field more than fifteen years ago were often trained with this approach. It doesn't necessarily mean that they're bad doctors, but you might not be comfortable with a physician who has this perspective. As we saw, Patricia ultimately did go to another doctor whose care satisfied her, but the entire episode was upsetting nonetheless.

Maura also felt caught between conflicting views. As she read and talked to her friends about hysterectomy, she was well aware of the controversy, but she still didn't know *how* those issues applied to her. As a result, she felt ambivalent about the operation, despite the fact that it clearly benefited her health.

At a time when there's such disagreement surrounding hysterectomies and when others' views can so strongly affect what a woman decides—not to mention how she feels about that decision—it is more essential than ever for a woman to make the effort to learn as much as she can about the operation. It's important to realize that there are real physical and emotional repercussions (if she's considering having a hysterectomy) and that (if she's already had one) the aftereffects she's experiencing are not simply her imagination. Often simply being prepared for what may unfold can help ease the adjustment, for depression and connected problems are frequently related to a sense of not having control over your life and health. Also, recognizing that you're not alone can greatly lessen the trauma.

Because we may well be in a phase of transition, when many of the myths among both medical consumers and medical providers are in the process of being corrected, it might be helpful to get some perspective on the controversy itself. Both the old, thankfully outdated, views about hysterectomy and the current response are factors in how women today experience and perceive their health. First, let's take a look at the historical picture.

While the first hysterectomy wasn't performed until 1853 (and it was still ten years before the first *successful* one), the notion of removing the uterus has a long and divisive history. The term "hysterectomy," in fact, comes from classical Greek: the word *hystera*, which means uterus or womb, and *ectomy*, from *ektemnein*, meaning to cut out or remove. In primitive and classical cultures the uterus was thought to be a separate entity—as Paula Weideger puts it in her book *History's Mistress*, "a kind of animal enclosed in the woman's body." It was thought that if no fertilization occurred at a given time, the uterus, disappointed and distraught, would wander about the body, stirring up fierce anxiety and disease in its restlessness. The uterus was considered to be a perpetual source of illness. Hence the pronouncement by Hippocrates, the Greek physician who is often called the father of medicine: "What is woman? Disease."

In the nineteenth century, too, the uterus was associated with a multitude of ills. The theory was that women, burdened by the presence of their reproductive organs, were bound to suffer from endless physical and emotional disturbances. The uterus and ovaries were said to "rule" the woman's body, subjugating her to the monthly periods that so weakened her. The added concern was that her tyrannical parts would render a woman "hysterical" (note the use again of *hystera*, the Greek term for uterus) when they grew too powerful to control. The uterus was assumed to be instrumental in all women's disorders, particularly emotional ones (which included, in this view, masturbating, expressing sexual desire, or deriving pleasure from intercourse—all of which "experts" of the period claimed would detract from a woman's health, sanity, and ability to conceive). That the repression of female sexuality and independence was a great—if not the greatest—cause of failing female health during this era would have to wait for later generations to discover.

It was during this period that gynecology as a specialty developed from the broader field of surgery. With the then prevalent emphasis on the female organs as the center of disease, the new group of specialists took every opportunity to "treat" the troublesome womb: shifting its position, injecting various compounds, and installing elaborate or unwieldy pessaries, which are instruments placed internally like a diaphragm in order to support a prolapsed, or fallen, uterus. In the 1870s, oophorectomies, or the removal of the ovaries, became popular operations and a decade later hysterectomies became common as well. The justification for them, however, was often suspect (unruly behavior, for instance) and the mortality rate incredibly high (as much as 40 percent in the early years of oophorectomies).

As it headed into the twentieth century, medical science made tremendous strides. The use of X rays, anesthesia, and antibiotics greatly enhanced the safety of surgical procedures. Using clean instruments and rubber gloves proved no less important to safe and successful surgery, since postoperative infections were a frequent cause of postsurgical complications and even death.

In many ways the stage had been set for the very conflicts faced today. As Barbara Ehrenreich and Deirdre English explain in their excellent discussion of women's relationship to the health care establishment, *For Her Own Good: One Hundred Fifty Years of Experts' Advice to Women*, physicians persisted in regarding the female reproductive organs as physical and emotional liabilities. Hysterectomies became increasingly common as doctors became more proficient at them, while they would brush aside women's doubts about hysterectomy by saying, "You'd be better off without it anyway." In the authors' words: "The female reproductive organs would continue to be viewed as a kind of frontier for chemical and surgical expansionism, untested drugs, and reckless experimentation."

As many surgical procedures became more routine, physicians in general seemed increasingly disposed to do them. In 1974 a Senate investigation into unnecessary surgery reported that there were 2.4 million unnecessary operations a year in this country.

Why is unnecessary surgery so pervasive? For one thing, medicine is a results-oriented profession, and a physician may lean toward surgery because it will clearly get results. Physicians tend to favor "definitive" solutions; in their view, doing their job successfully may mean taking definitive action to solve a problem—even if, in the case of hysterectomy, checking back periodically to see how a condition is progressing might in fact be preferable to surgery. Increased specialization in medicine is another factor. Doctors may be inclined to focus on ridding the patient of one problem instead of on exploring what's best in terms of her general health.

Some critics of medicine accuse doctors of greed, saying that doctors opt for the more lucrative procedure, as surgery frequently is. (A hysterectomy might cost anywhere from $2,000 to $5,000—and even higher in some urban areas.) They cite research showing that hysterectomies are more frequent when patients pay per procedure than when there is a one-time payment for services. Economics can work the other way as well. Some medical providers, such as health maintenance organizations (HMOs), may discourage their physicians from recommending tests or surgery because patients pay one fee regardless of what services they get. In such situations the question is whether the people who truly need certain types of surgery are receiving it.

Then there are the legal issues. Malpractice litigation, whether or not actual malpractice has occurred, is on the increase. Doctors may choose to do surgery to protect themselves. They are typically sued for failing to do something, not for doing "everything they could." So if a patient doesn't absolutely *need* a hysterectomy but the physician feels that the decision *not* to operate may come back to haunt him or her in the form of a lawsuit, the decision may be to operate. Obstetricians and gynecologic surgeons, in fact, have among the highest fees for malpractice insurance.

Of the ten most common surgical procedures, five are performed strictly on women: caesarean section; hysterectomy; dilation and curettage (D & C); bilateral destruction or occlusion (closure) of the fallopian tubes (for sterilization); and oophorectomy and salpingo-oophorectomy (excision of a fallopian tube and ovary). If this list doesn't indicate that gynecological patients bear the brunt of surgical excess, it at least suggests that with such operations so prevalent, patients are more likely to confront the possibility of surgery whose urgency is debatable.

According to Herbert H. Keyser, M.D., gynecologist and author of *Women Under the Knife*, women are particularly vulnerable to unnecessary surgery, which he calls "hazardous medicine." He cites a number of reasons, including the fact that women may feel intimidated by physicians, who are often male. Women sometimes tend to minimize their concerns when talking to their physicians and feel reluctant to question their judgment or request a second opinion. When you go for help to someone like a doctor, you are basically going to that person for a service. But on an emotional level you may feel you're putting him or her in a position of authority over you (and in many ways the medical profession perpetuates this view). It can be threatening to challenge those in power, for you may fear that by questioning you risk losing their support.

In the case of hysterectomy, Keyser adds that many women are anxious about contraception and believe the operation would free them from their worry about birth control. However, a tubal ligation is a much simpler means of sterilization. Hysterectomy for sterilization (hysterilization) does occur, even though most physicians feel that performing a hysterectomy chiefly for sterilization and without other medical reasons is unindicated.

Disturbingly, this seems to have been a particular problem among poor or minority women. Between 1970 and 1978 the hysterectomy rate for black women was much higher than that for white women. A separate study showed that poor women in public facilities are most prone to have hysterectomies. Part of this may reflect untreated medical conditions that required surgical treatment. Some critics, however, have pointed to the percentage of hysterectomies on poor and minority women done for sterilization, suggesting that hysterectomy for sterilization is a form of discrimination or social control. It's also worth noting that during periods when abortion services are curtailed, sterilization procedures become more available. With potential future changes in abortion laws, this may be worth monitoring closely.

However, many of the trends negatively affecting women's health seem to be changing. One major force countering them has been the women's movement: women have been learning more about their bodies and have been more demanding of rights. In terms of medicine, women have learned that many treatments offered up to them as cure-alls have turned out to have a darker side. The list includes intrauterine devices (IUDs), hormone treatments, and diethylstilbestrol (DES), which was prescribed in the 1950s and early 1960s to prevent miscarriage and was later found to cause a precancerous condition or actual cancer among a small percentage of the users' daughters (see Chapter 4, Cancer).

This awareness has encouraged women to be more discriminating medical consumers, but it has also led to a disillusionment with doctors—which can be unnerving to a woman who has no choice but to depend on doctors to some extent. No matter how well-read, no patient can have available to her all the information (clinical observations, test results, etc.) that her doctor would.

But information alone can make a huge difference, not only to the individual but to women as a group. A study in Switzerland found that after a public information campaign about hysterectomies in the mass media, the rate of operations dropped 25.8 percent. (The same study also found that female doctors performed about half as many hysterectomies as male doctors did—an interesting finding.)

There is no reason today for a woman to be a "victim" of medicine. Today's medical community is more receptive to women's concerns about hysterectomies, and if your doctor is not sensitive to your doubts and thinks you're being out of line in voicing them, it's your doctor— not you—who is at fault. Under such circumstances you should consider switching physicians, since you need, and deserve, medical care that addresses you as a whole person, not merely as an aggregate of body parts.

But it's important not to forget that, despite its controversial history, hysterectomy cannot be regarded as a weapon against women. It is an important surgical *tool* that, when properly indicated and properly performed, can be a tremendous boost to a woman's health. Although it's often the traumatic, troublesome, and needless operations that we most frequently hear about, as well we should, there are far greater numbers of women who are pleased with the results.

Janet's experience is probably typical: A forty-two-year-old businesswoman with one child, she was suffering from excessive bleeding—bleeding bad enough to leave her chronically weak and to lower her blood count significantly. It turned out that fibroids were the cause. Her doctor, a woman Janet felt she could talk to, told her she could have a hysterectomy or she could opt for a more conservative treatment, such as a myomectomy. The doctor explained that with a conservative alternative, there might yet be a need to do a hysterectomy later. Rarely can one procedure serve as a simple substitute for another.

Recently divorced, Janet wasn't expecting to have any more children—which would have been one reason to select a myomectomy instead—and she had the hysterectomy. After a month or two of recuperation, she felt terrific. Both her professional life and her home life improved, she said, because now she had the energy to tackle what she needed to do.

If, like Janet, you have an understanding of the operation and what it means, a clear sense of your own condition and needs, and are willing to work *with* your doctor (instead of simply being worked *on* by him or her), there is no reason for your own involvement with hysterectomy not to be a positive one.

CHAPTER 2

Hysterectomy and Related Operations

The word *hysterectomy* is defined as the surgical removal of the uterus. But the term, as commonly used, actually refers to several different operations, all of which involve removing the uterus. So before you get set for surgery, find out exactly what will be taken out. Some operations leave the cervix or the ovaries intact, for example, and for specific medical reasons this might be advised. Be sure that you have your terms straight. The phrase *partial hysterectomy*, often used by the lay public, may mean different things to different people. For example, leaving the ovaries in place while removing the uterus and cervix is actually termed a *total* hysterectomy as opposed to a partial one. To clear up some of the name confusion, here is a list of the various types of hysterectomies and a brief description of each:

1. *Total hysterectomy*. In this, by far the most common of the hysterectomy operations, the entire uterus is removed, including both the body and the neck (the cervix). Although often referred to as though it were a distinct organ, the cervix is technically a part of the uterus—the part that expands to let the baby come out during childbirth and that is generally extracted along with the body of the uterus. Hysterectomy puts a stop to menstrual periods and precludes any possibility of a woman's conceiving and bearing a child. Unless the ovaries are taken out, however, the monthly cyclic hormonal changes will continue.

2. *Supracervical hysterectomy* (sometimes called a "subtotal hysterectomy"). Here, the top of the uterus, or fundus, is taken out and the cervix is left in place. An advantage to this procedure, aside from its complying with a conservative approach of leaving the body alone as much as possible, is that some women experience a change in sexual function when the cervix is removed. One reason is that the nerves and blood vessels at the very top of the vagina are severed in total hysterectomy. And for some women, the sensation of the man's penis thrusting against the cervix is highly pleasurable. Also, in a total hysterectomy the vagina is sometimes shortened slightly, resulting in pain during intercourse for some women.

Another plus for the supracervical option is that because removing the cervix requires incisions quite close to the bladder and ureter, the chance of serious urinary complications is lower.

The downside is that when the cervix is left in, there's always a risk of cervical cancer (see Chapter 4, Cancer), and after a supracervical hysterectomy, treatment for cervical cancer becomes more difficult and possibly less effective. At that point treatment by hysterectomy or radical hysterectomy is no longer an option, and radiation treatment may have less effect. Whether or not the cervix is taken out, a regular Pap test is required. With the cervix removed, the Pap smear checks for cancer of the vagina, although it is extremely rare in women who have not had cancer or precancerous changes of the cervix. Those who have had these, or who have had a history of genital warts, or who have been exposed to DES in utero, are at a greater risk. Women who have had the cervix removed and have no other risk factors may have Pap tests less frequently, but such tests are still important.

In the early days of hysterectomies, the supracervical operation was usually performed because this procedure was thought to be easier. Then, with advances in surgical techniques, removing the entire uterus was deemed preferable, and the total hysterectomy was regarded as the standard. The supracervical procedure was reserved for cases where for various reasons the cervix proved difficult to extract or where the process of removing it increased risk of injury to surrounding organs. Still, many insurance companies today won't reimburse their subscribers for supracervical hysterectomies because they consider it to be an antiquated operation. Only in recent years has it been viewed as a routine option by physicians, largely because of the awareness of potential changes in sexual function. In Europe, where physicians tend to be less aggressive about surgery in general, the supracervical hysterectomy has become more common and is preferred by some physicians because of the reduced risk of injuring the ureter or bladder.

3. *Radical hysterectomy*. In this operation the entire uterus, including the cervix, the top portion of the vagina (sometimes called a "vaginal cuff"), and much of the tissue in the pelvic cavity that surrounds the cervix, called the parametrial tissue, is removed. Pelvic lymph nodes are frequently removed as well. A radical hysterectomy requires extensive surgery and therefore brings with it a greater risk of complications. The operation is usually called for in the case of cervical cancer or endometrial cancer that has spread to the cervix.

Today this operation is relatively rare. Because of frequent Pap smears, women with cervical cancer can generally be treated when the disease is less advanced and a less invasive procedure will suffice.

4. *Hysterectomy with bilateral salpingo-oophorectomy*. This term seems like a mouthful, but what it means, simply, is the removal of the uterus along with both ovaries and fallopian tubes. *Salpingo* refers to the fallopian tube (and derives from *salpinx,* the Greek word for trumpet), and *oophorectomy* means removal of the ovaries. Occasionally, only one tube and ovary are removed (unilateral salpingo-oophorectomy).

This operation is warranted when disease—such as cancer, severe infection, or severe endometriosis—has spread, and its control requires that these structures be removed. This would particularly apply to certain cases of a disorder like endometriosis, since the severity of discomfort is often related to ovarian hormone production.

In women who are approaching menopause or have completed it, the ovaries may be removed during a routine hysterectomy, to end any risk of ovarian cancer. For many years this was done virtually automatically. Today the ovaries are removed in perhaps half of hysterectomy patients over forty—even if the ovaries appear to be normal at the time of surgery. Overall, the ovaries are taken out in about 25 percent of all hysterectomies. The proportion of women having their ovaries and tubes removed at the time of hysterectomy appears to be highest in the northeastern states. As more is being learned about hormones and their interaction with the body even after natural menopause, this practice is being reevaluated. However, every woman must weigh the benefits of ovarian preservation with the risks of ovarian cancer, a disease which is difficult to detect in the early stages and which has a high mortality rate.

In almost all cases, the ovary and fallopian tube are taken out together, chiefly because they lie so close together in the pelvic cavity as to almost be attached. Each ovary shares the blood supply with its corresponding tube, so attempting to remove one without the other can interfere with blood flow.

Particularly with younger women, who would be jolted into menopause if both ovaries were taken out, it is often beneficial to leave in at least one ovary and fallopian tube, if possible. This will preserve ovarian function and thus maintain the level of hormones produced by the ovaries. When there's a benign cyst on one ovary, for example, and the other ovary is normal, the unaffected ovary and tube may be left intact. Even after a hysterectomy, women with ovaries left in place should have a pelvic exam at least once a year.

5. *Caesarean hysterectomy.* This is when the uterus is taken out immediately after a baby is delivered through an abdominal incision. This rare procedure is usually resorted to under two conditions. One is if the mother has been diagnosed with cancer in the pelvic region (for example, cancer of the cervix), and in this way the baby is delivered and the mother is treated for disease at the same time.

The other condition is when uncontrolled bleeding occurs during a caesarean delivery. The hysterectomy is done to save the mother from excessive, possibly life-threatening blood loss. Unfortunately, the mother has no choice in this situation, though she will not be able to conceive again.

Physically, this is quite a stressful operation because it's really two separate operations performed simultaneously. As a result, the risk of complications is high and the recovery time fairly long. Also, because blood vessels are dilated during pregnancy, the potential for blood loss is much greater.

There are two basic methods of hysterectomy: vaginal and abdominal. One or the other may be recommended because of the specific conditions that have led to hysterectomy; the patient's age and relative health (and thus susceptibility to surgical complications); and the doctor's particular skill and experience (he or she may be more proficient in or comfortable with one type). If you have any question as to which is best for you, consider getting a second opinion.

In a *vaginal* hysterectomy the entire uterus is removed through the opening in the vagina. This approach is most commonly used when the uterus has fallen, or prolapsed, and when vaginal repairs, such as tightening muscles that have relaxed in the process of childbirth, are needed. Because the uterus itself must be removed from bottom to top, it's not possible to do a supracervical hysterectomy this way. Nor is a vaginal hysterectomy appropriate in most cases of cancer, when the uterus is significantly enlarged (as it may be with fibroids), or when previous surgery or a condition such as endometriosis has left scar tissue in the pelvic area. Because physicians are becoming increasingly conservative about doing surgery and are waiting until the indications for hysterectomy are more clear (often until a later point when conditions may preclude vaginal hysterectomy), fewer are being done.

About 25 percent of hysterectomies among premenopausal women are done vaginally. The proportion among women forty-five and older is higher, since uterine prolapse (the falling of the uterus) tends to occur later in life. For some reason the rate of hysterectomies performed vaginally seems to be highest in the western United States and lowest in the Northeast. This is generally the preferred procedure with elderly women or those with a heart condition, who may be at greater risk with the more intrusive abdominal method.

In this operation, the vagina is stretched by using special instruments to keep it open. The uterus is removed after clamping, cutting, and tying off the blood vessels and ligaments that connect it to the body.

The advantage of the vaginal hysterectomy is that there's no abdominal incision. The cut is made through the top of the vagina, at the cervix, and there will be no visible scar afterward. If the operation proceeds without complication, the hospital stay may well be shorter and the return of bowel function quicker. There will also be less abdominal pain because there has been no abdominal cut.

Some women, however, get backaches for a short time after the operation, primarily because during the procedure they have been positioned on their backs with their legs up for an extended period. The ovaries may or may not be removed with a vaginal hysterectomy, but since it's more difficult to take them out with this method, they are often left in place.

Often the vaginal hysterectomy is performed in conjunction with repair of the bladder and rectum, which will probably prolong recuperation time a bit. Also, there may be instances when bleeding from the blood vessels occurs as the surgeon is clamping them off, and then a switch to an abdominal incision may be necessary.

One drawback to the vaginal approach is the evidence that it is more likely to impair sexual function. When the hysterectomy is done to correct a prolapse, for example, the vagina may be tightened or shortened to a point where intercourse is difficult or even painful.

In an *abdominal* hysterectomy, the most frequent method, the uterus is removed through a surgical incision of about six to eight inches in the lower abdomen. Two significant cuts are required during the operation: the initial abdominal cut to gain access to the pelvic cavity (which actually goes through several layers of tissue), and the subsequent cut at the vagina to detach the uterus. It is considered the optimal procedure to employ when the ovaries will be taken out or when disease has spread to the pelvic cavity. It's also usually used for women who have had previous abdominal or pelvic surgery. With this technique the surgeon is in a better position to explore internally, so it's generally selected in instances of any undiagnosed problems, or when there may be adhesions in the pelvic area as a result of previous operations, endometriosis, or infection.

Because of the abdominal incision, however, the recovery period is usually longer and certain movements or tasks may cause discomfort. The complication rate is also reported to be anywhere from two to four times higher than that of vaginal hysterectomies.

As in the vaginal hysterectomy, the dissection involves careful clamping, cutting, and tying. But here, a second incision is made in the vagina in order to detach the uterus. Then the top of the vagina and later the abdominal incision (in many layers) are closed.

The surgeon will either make a vertical cut, or a horizontal cut—often referred to as a "bikini cut." The up-and-down incision starts at about the navel and extends down to the pubic bone. It is usually preferred when there's any chance of cancer, so that tissue in the upper abdominal region can be examined and biopsied if there is reason to believe the disease has spread. Because the vertical incision provides more room, it is often chosen when the uterus is enlarged or when there are sizable ovarian cysts.

The bikini cut, which runs along the top of the pubic-hair line, is more common in the case of benign disease. It is often chosen for cosmetic reasons (the scar that results from the straight-across cut is less visible), and some physicians feel it makes for a stronger incision with greater abdominal support. Because many doctors have their own preferences, however, it would be a good idea to inquire about which procedure yours is planning to do.

Of the number of related tests and procedures that are generally done before surgery, some of the most common include:

1. *The Pap smear*. This is to test for cancer of the cervix and other cervical disorders. This simple procedure, which involves collecting a scraping of cells from the surface of the cervix and then examining the sample in a laboratory to search out any abnormalities, is regularly conducted in a gynecologist's office during routine pelvic exams. It is generally recommended that women have the test every year, since early indications for cervical cancer can develop during a twelve-month interval, and the quicker the disease is caught, the better. Women who are thought to be at a higher risk for cervical cancer should be tested more frequently.

An abnormal reading on a Pap test by no means suggests that you're destined for a hysterectomy. It merely notes that there are abnormal cells (possibly precancerous or inflammatory) in the cervix. At one time hysterectomies were done on the basis of an abnormal Pap test alone, but today precancerous conditions in the cervix or even early forms of cervical cancer are often treated by less radical measures. Monitoring the conditions with Pap smears and colposcopy (magnified examination with a speculum inserted in the vagina) and treating them as they arise greatly lessen the chances of needing a hysterectomy later on (see Chapter 4, Cancer).

A Pap smear should precede every hysterectomy, to check for undiagnosed cervical cancer. At an advanced state, invasive cervical cancer is often treated by radiation therapy or radical hysterectomy. If such a cancer is indeed found, a simple hysterectomy would be the absolutely wrong medical choice.

2. *D & C*. A D & C ("dilation and curettage") is a scraping of the uterine lining. It might be used in diagnosis, to obtain a tissue sample for possible cancerous or precancerous conditions or to determine the cause of excessive uterine bleeding. In other cases it might be used to remove polyps or overgrown tissue from the uterine wall, a procedure that could then treat the cause of uncontrolled bleeding. In this way a D & C may preclude the need for a hysterectomy. A D & C might be done prior to a scheduled hysterectomy to insure there's no cancer present, because a malignancy might require treatment other than a hysterectomy. Other common uses for D & C's are to terminate an unwanted pregnancy and to remove any tissue remaining following delivery of a baby, a miscarriage, or an incomplete abortion.

The procedure is usually done in the hospital under a general or local anesthetic. Using dilators of increasing sizes, the doctor will widen the opening of the cervix and then scrape the uterine lining with a narrow curette. The tissue removed will be saved for examination. After a D & C, the patient can usually return home the same day.

3. *Cone biopsy of the cervix*. In this procedure, usually done in the hospital on an out-patient basis under general or local anesthesia, a cone-shaped wedge of tissue is removed from the cervix using either a scalpel or a laser. Some physicians feel that the laser cone results in less scarring and less bleeding than the scalpel method. There are reservations about its use, however, since some experts believe that the laser disturbs the specimen sent to the pathology laboratory, and therefore may produce false or misleading results.

The cone biopsy is diagnostic, to determine the depth and possible invasion of abnormal cells. If the cone reveals a spreading malignancy, treatment such as a radical hysterectomy may be needed. The cone biopsy can, in many cases, also be therapeutic; for example, when a precancerous condition turns out to be well contained, simply removing the abnormal cells may be sufficient treatment.

Many cases now handled by cone biopsy would have been traditionally treated with hysterectomy. One reason to be wary about cone biopsies, however, is that in some cases, if the cone biopsy is taken very deep into the cervix or if the cervix is structurally abnormal (as in some women who have been exposed to DES), it could compromise fertility or induce difficulty in childbirth. Studies have refuted this allegation, but if you do wish to have children, it may be wise to discuss this with your doctor and perhaps ask whether the area that must be removed may cause such problems.

One relatively recent variation on the cone biopsy that is gaining in prevalence is a laser ablation cone. Instead of the cone's being removed and sent to a lab for examination, the tissue is simply vaporized. This operation is far easier to do than a laser excisional cone and can be performed as an office procedure with a local anesthetic or no anesthetic at all. But it's appropriate only in cases where the depth and extent of the abnormal cells are known and have been confirmed by previous biopsies.

4. *Laparoscopy*. This procedure, like the cone biopsy and the D & C, is used for both diagnostic and curative purposes, in this case for pelvic pain or endometriosis. The doctor inserts a thin tube—almost like a needle— through a tiny incision in the abdomen near the belly button. Gas is blown in through the tube to inflate the abdomen. Then a light-emitting scope is placed through the same incision so that the pelvic and abdominal organs can be looked at directly.

With the laparoscope, the doctor can examine the pelvic organs. The test often gives the doctor information unattainable by other methods, such as X ray or ultrasound. Scar tissue resulting from pelvic inflammatory disease or endometriosis may be diagnosed in this way.

A cautery or a laser can be used along with the laparoscope to cut or remove pelvic adhesions. The procedure has a number of other applications: for diagnosing and treating infertility, endometriosis, or ectopic pregnancy, or for tubal sterilization. More and more surgical procedures are being done this way, but for many conditions related to hysterectomy, such as large fibroids and most instances of cancer, the laparoscope is of little use.

Laparoscopy is typically done under a general anesthetic, and the entire process takes as little as an hour if it's for diagnostic purposes only, but up to four hours if there is treatment as well.

CHAPTER 3

Fibroids

In the United States today, more hysterectomies are done because of fibroids than for any other reason, accounting for at least one fourth of all those performed. Fibroids, or uterine leiomyomas, are lumps of tissue that originate in the muscle of the uterine wall (the myometrium). Despite their being technically tumors, a word we often associate with malignancy, fibroids are almost always benign (fewer than 1 percent prove to be cancerous). The trouble with fibroids is that they can grow so large that they start pressing down on other organs, such as the bladder or the bowel, and, depending on their size and location, can cause other uncomfortable symptoms, among them heavy bleeding and pelvic pain.

If your doctor suspects fibroids, he or she may order a sonogram. This test, which is based on sound waves, is also commonly performed during pregnancy. Here it is done to determine the size and location of the fibroids, and serves to confirm whether the mass discovered is indeed one fibroid or many fibroids. Occasionally other conditions, such as ovarian tumors, feel very much like fibroids on examination.

Regular X rays don't reveal fibroids. Magnetic resonance imaging (MRI), which uses radio waves, may occasionally be ordered if there's a difficult diagnosis or suspicion of malignancy.

A diagnosis of fibroids does not necessarily mean there's a hysterectomy in your future. There are alternative treatments, and if the fibroids cause no discomfort—and are not growing rapidly—the treatment of choice may be to do nothing at all.

It is estimated that between 20 percent and 25 percent of all women of reproductive age develop fibroids. Some experts put that estimate even higher, because many women won't even know they have them. Fibroids can grow anywhere within the uterus or extending from the uterus. Those that develop on the inside of the uterus are called "submucous fibroids"; those growing on the outside are termed "subserous fibroids." A third type, "intramural fibroids," are found within the walls of the uterus. Subserous and intramural fibroids tend not to cause problems unless they are very large and begin to exert pressure on other organs. Even small submucous fibroids, however, can cause heavy bleeding and fertility problems.

Women may have one fibroid or several. The tumors can be quite small or they can weigh in at several pounds. Many gynecologists consider a fibroid that has grown to the size of a three-month pregnancy cause for hysterectomy. Others, however, argue that many women with large—even very large—fibroids are not uncomfortable, so size alone rarely justifies operating.

Fibroids usually grow fairly slowly. Sometimes the pattern is that they grow in spurts, and for long periods there may be little or no gain in size. A fibroid that's growing quite rapidly could be a sign of malignancy, but, as noted before, the chances of a fibroid being malignant are slight.

What causes fibroids to grow is not clear. They seem to be related to hormones, particularly estrogen, but also growth hormone and progesterone. For this reason, estrogen replacement therapy or other hormonal medications including birth control pills may promote their growth. Alert your physician if this is the case. Fibroids grow during pregnancy (when hormone levels are particularly high) and shrink as menopause approaches and ensues. For this reason, women who develop fibroids close to menopause are often advised to stick it out because the fibroids will soon subside on their own.

The side effects of fibroids, when they occur, vary greatly. Between 50 percent and 80 percent are estimated to produce no symptoms at all. About one third of all women whose fibroids do cause symptoms have heavy bleeding, between periods as well as during them. Occasionally fibroids cause infertility, although factors besides fibroids may also contribute to this. Because fibroids tend to develop toward the end of a woman's reproductive life, and because the trend is to choose to have children later, this may be of increasing concern. Hysterectomy, of course, may take care of the fibroids, but it is no solution to the problem of infertility. However, myomectomy, discussed later in this chapter, is often used effectively to remove fibroids while preserving fertility, as are combined treatments of drugs and myomectomy. Other complications of pregnancy, such as spontaneous abortion, can sometimes be linked to fibroids as well.

Pelvic pain or pressure are also symptoms associated with fibroids. A woman with fibroids may experience no more than a bloated or full feeling (and may notice that her clothes are fitting tighter), or she may have severe pain. Large fibroids may also cause problems by putting pressure on other organs in the pelvic cavity, including the bladder, bowel, and rectum. Usually the effects are fairly minor—for instance, urinary frequency or bowel pressure—but more severe obstruction does occasionally occur. Bleeding can result if fibroids develop deep in the lining of the uterus. This, in fact, is the most common cause of surgery for the condition. Fibroids can also cause discomfort during sexual intercourse.

HOW DOES A HYSTERECTOMY HELP?

When fibroids cause trouble, one clear solution is hysterectomy. A hysterectomy should ease any unpleasant symptoms of fibroids. The fibroids and the site of their growth are removed, so there is no chance of their growing back. It is important, however, that you rule out any other possible causes of the symptoms, for pelvic pressure or abnormal bleeding can occur for a number of reasons. Unless the fibroid is malignant, there is no urgent need for a hysterectomy, so you should take the time to explore other courses of treatment. With a malignancy, however, a hysterectomy is the only option and should be planned immediately.

ALTERNATIVE TREATMENTS

One alternative to hysterectomy is an operation called a "myomectomy." This is a surgical removal of uterine fibroids. Like hysterectomy, this is major surgery requiring a minimum of five days in the hospital, but in a myomectomy the uterus is repaired rather than removed. The chief advantage is that the uterus and ovaries—and thus fertility—are unaffected.

It's possible that scar tissue formed as a result of the operation may itself compromise fertility. But it certainly gives you more than the zero chance of having a baby that a hysterectomy would. Of women who want children, more than half prove able to conceive after undergoing a myomectomy, and the rate of spontaneous abortion is only slightly higher in this group than in the population at large.

Following a myomectomy, particularly if the fibroids were removed from deep inside the uterine wall, a woman may be urged to give birth by caesarean section. That's because the procedure could leave the uterus in a weaker state, raising the possibility of uterine rupture during vaginal delivery. The downside of myomectomy is that since the operation is a fairly complex one, in which the uterus is virtually taken apart (to remove the fibroids) then sewn back together, there's a greater chance of complication during the postoperative period. Postoperative problems could include bleeding, infection, and interference with bowel function. Bleeding can become heavy, and the chances of requiring a transfusion are much greater in a myomectomy than with hysterectomy. Occasionally, though rarely, the bleeding at the time of operating is so profuse that the surgeon may need to switch and perform a hysterectomy on the spot in order to control it.

Nor is myomectomy always an option, often depending on the size and position of the fibroids. If the fibroids have gotten particularly large, for example, it might not be possible to remove them without extracting the entire uterus. And if there are numerous small fibroids, for instance, fifty, it may prove too difficult to take them all out.

If you decide to have a myomectomy, it's important that your doctor know your feelings regarding hysterectomy. Ultrasound can give the doctor some information about the size and whereabouts of the tumors, but often he or she cannot have anticipated your condition until you've been opened up. Some fibroids may be especially difficult to reach, so that a hysterectomy may have to be done after all in order to remove them.

Also, with the uterus still intact the fibroids may recur after the operation, as they do in about 10 percent to 20 percent of women who have had myomectomies. Fibroids close to the uterus's outer surface or actually within the wall tend to be less likely to recur. It is possible to repeat the procedure—several times, even—

but subsequent operations may be more difficult if adhesions have developed.

Many physicians are reluctant to perform myomectomies. A doctor who is not very comfortable with the procedure may try to discourage you from having it done, perhaps insisting that you have too many fibroids or that they've grown too large. (While this may indeed be true for this particular doctor, there may be other physicians who would have no qualms about proceeding with the operation. Do get a second opinion if you suspect this is the case.) Technically, it's not a terribly arduous operation, but it can be messy and doing a thorough job of removing the tumors can take a long time.

Until recently, myomectomies were nearly unheard of in this country. If they were done at all, it was strictly for women who specifically wished to have more children. Fortunately, the value of the uterus, aside from its function in childbearing, is becoming appreciated. Today, the procedure is becoming more current in the United States (as it long has been in Europe), affording another option to women who want to retain their reproductive organs. A myomectomy will probably cost about the same as a hysterectomy, but the insurance company may reimburse you at a lower rate. This is in part because the operation is still in the process of gaining widespread acceptance.

A thirty-eight-year-old woman with two children, Nancy was found to have a fibroid the size equivalent of a four-and-a-half-month pregnancy. Her doctor said it was too large for a myomectomy and recommended a hysterectomy. Although she didn't plan to have any additional children, she wanted at least to have the option—which the hysterectomy wouldn't give her. So she spoke to a doctor friend and found a second physician who regularly performed myomectomies, and had the fibroid removed this way.

Myomectomies are generally done with a scalpel, but they can also be performed with a laser. Some doctors feel that patients lose less blood with a laser, but it's not clear whether a laser indeed provides an advantage.

A variation on the standard abdominal myomectomy is a vaginal myomectomy. Occasionally a submucous myoma is present on a stalk protruding through the cervix and can be removed vaginally simply by clamping off the base of the stalk. Also, small submucous fibroids can sometimes be extracted through a hysteroscope, using a cautery or a laser. An advantage to this is that there's no abdominal incision. Only a small percentage of fibroids may be removed this way, however. It's also possible to remove fibroids on the outside of the uterus using a laparoscope and laser or cautery, but again this may be done only in select cases, and only if the fibroids are small.

Drug treatments can also aid in controlling fibroids. Some doctors have tried using a type of drug called "GnRH analogs," which create an artificial menopause, or Danocrine, a drug often used to treat endometriosis. At this point neither drug has been FDA-approved for controlling fibroids. (Lupron GnRH serves as treatment for prostate cancer.) Lupron is taken by a daily injection. Some women may initially find this a drawback, but it's usually not much trouble to learn (just as diabetics learn to give themselves daily insulin injections). A once-a-month injection form of this drug has been developed to eliminate the need for a daily injection, and an even newer drug, which is given as a nasal spray, has just been released.

Studies have attested to the effectiveness of such drugs, but patients on these treatments might not be reimbursed by insurance companies. Also, it's important to note that because certain drugs may propel you into menopause, other problems related to menopause—hot flashes, vaginal dryness, increased risk of osteoporosis—may arise.

Further, it is not advisable to take such drugs over a prolonged period of time because the hormonal shifts, especially the drop in estrogen, can cause other problems (see Chapter 12, The Question of Hormone Therapy). For this reason, drug therapy combined with other treatment, such as myomectomy, laparoscopy, or watchful waiting, would be best. An example would be to use drug treatments to shrink the fibroids until they're at a size where surgery is manageable. This would actually open up the possibility of myomectomy to women with large fibroids, who in the past could only have been treated with hysterectomy.

The other, less dramatic option is simply to wait and see what happens. If the fibroids cause no symptoms and are not large enough to present a threat to fertility, there's nothing that urgently needs to be done. This could be the best option for a woman who is nearing menopause and has only small or moderate-sized fibroids and suffers no severe symptoms.

WHEN IS A HYSTERECTOMY A GOOD IDEA?

If you have fibroids, is a hysterectomy the answer for you? Rarely is this clear. Fibroids are hardly ever a life-or-death condition. The mere thought of having a tumor or of carrying a growth that's as large as a three-month old fetus (which has traditionally been the arbitrary cutoff in size, despite the fact that many women do not have symptoms at this point) should not frighten you into agreeing to a hysterectomy. Do your fibroids bother you, or don't they? Would your level of comfort and quality of life improve once they're taken out? Are there any other ways to control them that might be better for your overall health? Are you close to menopause and, if so, is there a way to keep your fibroids manageable until such time when they recede on their own? Do you want to have children? These are the kinds of questions you should ask yourself—and the issues you need to raise with your doctor.

CHAPTER 4

Cancer

Approximately 10 percent of all hysterectomies are performed to treat cancer. These are the most clear-cut cases for hysterectomy; if cancer has developed in a woman's cervix, uterus, or ovaries, a hysterectomy could save her life and thus all other considerations would be secondary.

When the malignancy has not spread, the advantage of hysterectomy is that the region containing the cancer is removed, leaving the body free of disease. If the cancer is at the stage where it has extended to other areas, including the pelvic lymph nodes (because of the role of lymph fluid in carrying white blood cells to combat disease, cancer often initially spreads to the nodes), the bladder, and the bowel, other treatment may be needed instead of or in addition to hysterectomy. Hysterectomies may also be done to manage the spread of other cancers, such as cancer of the colon.

While a full-blown case of cancer leaves little choice but to operate, there are precancerous conditions that are less definite indicators for hysterectomy. This is where you have to decide whether there are other means of controlling any abnormal growth in cells that would be better suited to someone of your age, life-style, and relative health.

The very word *cancer* is bound to arouse fear in anyone—not to mention the thought of actually carrying any cancer in one's body. It's often assumed that hearing that you have cancer is a death sentence—a curtain drawn—and fears associated with cancer may cloud your thinking when it comes to making choices based on such a diagnosis.

But such news doesn't always herald a gloomy end. With great strides in the prevention, detection, and treatment of cancers, people are living longer—and better—well after the diagnosis is made. In the case of cervical, endometrial, and ovarian cancers, the five-year survival rate has been steadily climbing over the last several years. According to the American Cancer Society, the overall death rate from cervical and endometrial cancer has dropped more than 70 percent in the last forty years. The most important factor here is that women are having more frequent checkups and tests, so that the disease is caught at an early stage where the treatment success rate approaches 100 percent.

It's also important to note that daughters of women who were given DES (diethylstilbestrol, a drug at one time thought to prevent miscarriages and commonly prescribed to women up until the 1960s) are at an increased risk of developing a rare form of cancer of either the vagina or the cervix. Women who were exposed to the drug in utero should be absolutely sure to be closely monitored by twice-yearly examinations.

An abdominal hysterectomy will almost always be performed for treatment of cancer. This allows the surgeon to determine whether there has been any spread of disease to organs in the pelvis or abdomen, and to take biopsies or remove those organs if need demands. The incision used will nearly always be the vertical cut as opposed to the bikini cut, so that the entire region from the upper abdomen to the pelvis will be accessible.

CANCER OF THE CERVIX

This cancer occurs when the cells in the cervix change and become malignant. In the cervix, which is the end of the uterus that extends into the vagina, there are two types of tissue: tissue lining the cervical canal and tissue covering the outside of the cervix. At the point where they meet, the cells are constantly growing and replacing themselves, and it is at this point where abnormal growth most commonly begins.

The Pap test your gynecologist regularly gives you detects whether any abnormal cells are present. It is recommended Pap smears be taken every year once you become sexually active. Some authorities believe that if three consecutive years go by with no abnormalities, they can be done less frequently. Many others argue that they should always be done annually. If a hysterectomy is performed for precancerous or cancerous cellular changes in the cervix, regular Pap smears must still be done because cancer may occur in the vagina as well.

The Pap is only a screening test, however. After an abnormal Pap test, further examination is needed before a conclusive diagnosis can be made. For this a colposcopy may be done. Here the doctor looks through a colposcope for a magnified view of the vagina, cervix, and vulva. This visual exam can sometimes reveal the development of disease. Then biopsies are taken of the area that cannot be seen and of any abnormal areas. If abnormal cells are present but it is not clear whether they are invasive, a cone biopsy may be necessary. (In the past, before colposcopies were widely available, a cone was automatically ordered after any abnormal Pap smear.) If invasion has not occurred, and all abnormal cells have been removed by the cone biopsy with a margin of normal tissue, no further surgery may be necessary.

Pap smears are invaluable because symptoms often don't reveal themselves until the disease is well on its way. Bleeding after intercourse can be an early sign of disease. The chief risk factors for cervical cancer are intercourse at an early age and having multiple sex partners. There are theories, in fact, that cancer of the cervix is a sexually transmitted disease and related to sexually transmitted viruses. Carcinoma in situ of the cervix occurs when the abnormal cells are limited to the superficial layer of the cervix but have not yet invaded the deeper cervical tissue. This is a *pre*cancerous condition. It is nearly always curable and can usually be taken care of without a hysterectomy. (In the past, however, the uterus was removed at any hint of abnormal cells.) Dysplasia is a precursor to this stage. It is essential to begin treating any abnormal change in cells as soon as it's discovered. The progression of the disease is generally very slow, but in some instances the cells grow quite rapidly.

One alternative treatment for cervical dysplasia is cryosurgery. This can be done in a doctor's office and no anesthesia is needed. A probe is placed over the area of abnormal cells, and the tissue is destroyed by freezing. Laser treatment, where the affected tissue is vaporized, is another effective method. Whatever procedure is used, it is important to follow it up with frequent Pap smears to insure that no abnormal tissue was left in the body and that none has grown back.

Five years ago Julia was diagnosed with carcinoma in situ of the cervix and was told she should have a hysterectomy once she'd completed her family. Now thirty-four, Julia went back to her doctor. When a cone biopsy revealed that the condition was contained and the margins clear, the doctor told her she didn't need a hysterectomy but "we can follow you."

With Pap smears twice a year and a colposcopy if any abnormal cells are detected, women in Julia's situation can often be spared hysterectomy. It was previously thought that anyone diagnosed with carcinoma in situ of the cervix would ultimately develop cancer, that the treatment was merely putting the disease on hold. Studies have shown, however, that if the area of abnormal cells is completely removed and the margins are clear, the chances of developing further cancer in situ of the cervix are no greater than those of developing cancer in situ of the vagina if a hysterectomy has been performed.

Invasive cancer of the cervix is when the cancer has begun to spread. This is a potentially life-threatening condition and there should be no delay in taking action. Very early cases, when the spread has been contained to a minimal depth, are termed "microinvasion." Such cases must be treated on an individual basis, depending on the size of the abnormal cell area and the degree of invasion. Usually more than a simple hysterectomy is required with invasive cancer of the cervix, although the ovaries won't necessarily need to be taken out. For cervical cancer that has indeed begun to creep into the cervix, a radical hysterectomy or radiation treatment may be the treatment of choice.

CANCER OF THE ENDOMETRIUM

This refers to a cancer that develops in the lining of the uterus. It is also called cancer of the uterus. Postmenopausal women are most commonly afflicted with endometrial cancer, with the diagnosis most often occurring between ages fifty-five and sixty-nine. A number of risk factors that could signal a higher than usual chance of getting the disease include: a history of infertility; obesity; prolonged estrogen therapy (without progesterone); high blood pressure; diabetes; and a family history of endometrial cancer.

Abnormal bleeding is a frequent symptom, occurring in about 80 percent of cases. Any postmenopausal abnormal bleeding should be reported to your doctor. One problem with endometrial cancer, however, is that it's not always easy to diagnose. Although intended to diagnose cancer of the cervix, Pap smears will detect endometrial cancer about 50 percent of the time. Usually a D & C or an aspiration curettage (which is similar to a D & C but extracts a smaller sample and can be done in a doctor's office) is used to determine if cancer is present. Anyone who has abnormal bleeding after menopause should see her physician so that appropriate endometrial tissue samples can be taken.

A condition called "endometrial hyperplasia" generally precedes actual cancer of the endometrium. Excessive or unusual bleeding is the frequent symptom (see Chapter 6, Heavy Bleeding, Chronic Pain). This may occur because of abnormal hormone balances, such as those that occur with recurrent cycles in which ovulation does not take place. In such anovulatory cycles, the estrogen that is normally produced is not balanced by progesterone that would have been produced by the ovary after ovulation. Hyperplasias fall into different categories, with different precancerous potential. For example, benign cystic hyperplasia would be one of the least worrisome categories, and atypical adenomatous hyperplasia would be one of the worst.

In some cases where hyperplasia occurs, some treatments short of hysterectomy, such as administering high doses of progesterone, can still effectively cure the condition. However, in some cases of adenomatous or atypical adenomatous hyperplasia (when the condition is more advanced), this is not advisable. If the patient is past menopause when adenomatous hyperplasia develops, a hysterectomy is usually recommended.

If the disease has reached the point of invasive cancer of the endometrium, a hysterectomy will have to be done. A cancer confined to the uterus will be treated by a hysterectomy with the ovaries and both fallopian tubes removed. (Because endometrial cancer has a hormonal component the ovaries will always be removed.) At the time of the incision, more biopsies will be taken, perhaps from the lymph nodes and the omentum, the fold that hangs down from the intestine, to search for any possible microscopic spread of the disease.

If the cancer has spread, a hysterectomy may be done in conjunction with radiation, chemotherapy, or hormone treatment. These alone, however, cannot serve as a substitute for surgery. Radiation, for instance, has a much lower rate of curing the cancer.

Most women who have had a hysterectomy for uterine cancer are not able to take estrogen replacement therapy.

CANCER OF THE OVARY

Although cancer of the ovary is less common than either cervical or endometrial cancer, it causes more deaths than those two cancers combined. According to the American Cancer Society, about one out of every

seventy newborn girls will develop ovarian cancer during her lifetime.

Ovarian cancer is often described as "silent" because
there might be no symptoms until its later stages. There
may be no impairment of ovarian function until the
disease is quite advanced. Some signs that could
suggest ovarian cancer are lower abdominal pain and
an enlarged abdomen, which could be caused by the
collection of fluid. In women approaching or past menopause, any unexplained digestive disturbances (dis-
tension, gas, etc.) should probably be checked thoroughly to eliminate the possibility that ovarian cancer is
the cause.

The risk for cancer of the ovary rises with age, and
the chances of contracting it are highest in women aged
sixty-five to eighty-four. Women who have never had
children are twice as likely to get it, as are women
who have had breast cancer or endometrial cancer.
There also seems to be a tendency for it to run in
families.

Having a cyst or growth (other words you may hear
are *tumor, mass, thickness,* or *lump*) on the ovary does
not mean you have ovarian cancer. Benign (noncancer-
ous) cysts on the ovary do develop as well—indeed,
most cysts on the ovary are benign. Normal (functional)
cysts often occur as a result of the normal mechanism of
ovulation. If such cysts grow large or fail to go away (as
they generally do after a menstrual cycle), your doctor
may decide to operate. In part this is because doctors
cannot always tell whether there's a malignancy unless
they operate, and also because there may be a chance

that the cyst will rupture or cause other problems. With any cyst that develops after menopause, however, malignancy must be ruled out.

If your doctor tells you that you need surgery, make certain you know the reason for the operation. Does he or she suspect malignancy? (The chances of this are lower the younger you are.) Are there ways other than operating to determine whether the cyst is malignant? If you plan to have children, is there a chance that surgery will affect your ability to conceive? (The scar tissue that could result may interfere with fertility.) Are there any other options? (Sometimes a benign cyst can be removed without taking out the ovary.) Are there any circumstances under which your doctor would perform a hysterectomy?

It's important to have such issues clarified. If you do not want to have a nondiseased ovary removed simply because you're already opened up and because there's a chance it may someday become diseased, say so. Some women might state a wish to have a hysterectomy done under these circumstances. This might be the case if they have other pathology or discomfort, like painful, heavy bleeding, and this would be a way to have one operation instead of two.

Borderline ovarian tumors, which may have some of the characteristics of a malignancy but cannot conclusively be called cancer, are more common in premenopausal women. Because this is a precancerous condition that threatens to develop into ovarian cancer, and because ovarian cancer is both so virulent and so difficult to monitor, in many cases a hysterectomy is done. In some cases, however, to allow for having children, the doctor can remove strictly the affected ovary as well as taking many biopsies to make sure there is no evidence of malignancy in other areas. After this type of surgery, a patient will be followed closely for any signs of malignancy. In the case of borderline pathology, it's probably best to obtain a second opinion and to consult a cancer specialist.

Growths on the ovary are generally detected during a pelvic exam. (This is why routine gynecologist appointments are absolutely essential!) Pap smears are useless in detecting ovarian cancer. If a cyst is discovered, it needs to be examined to see if it's cancerous. Further information can be obtained by laparoscopy, ultrasound, or X ray, but often it is necessary to operate. During the actual surgery, tissue from the tumor may be sent to the lab for a frozen biopsy, one way of checking for malignancy. The visual examination can be revealing too. It's important that both ovaries are checked, because if one ovary is affected, disease may also be present in the other ovary.

If the existence of cancer has been established, the usual surgical treatment includes removing both ovaries, both fallopian tubes, and the uterus. If the cancer has advanced, an effort will be made to remove other affected tissue. Radiation therapy and drug therapy may be done in addition to surgery if the cancer has spread.

CHAPTER 5

Endometriosis

The pain from endometriosis has propelled many women to the operating room for treatment by hysterectomy. About 15 percent of all hysterectomies done are because of endometriosis, and many who seek surgery for this reason are young women still in the middle of their reproductive years. The proportion of hysterectomies performed for endometriosis is increasing, but so is the number of diagnosed cases.

The name of the disease refers to the endometrium, the tissue that lines the inside wall of the uterus and is shed each month through menstruation. In endometriosis, endometrium-like tissue crops up elsewhere in the body, attaching itself to other organs in the pelvic cavity. The growths are usually not malignant. But these endometrial implants *act* as if they were part of the uterine lining. As a result, they respond to hormones and build up and bleed in accordance with the menstrual cycle.

Because such activity is triggered by hormones, menopause generally eases the symptoms, as does pregnancy.

This internal bleeding can cause inflammation in the
areas it affects, and scar tissue usually develops. Sometimes self-protective cysts grow over the misplaced endometrial tissue and may swell, causing pain. Such
cysts, though benign, are apt to burst, setting off an
abnormal release of dark brown blood. This, too, can be
extremely painful. In response to the inflammation of
tissue and growth of cysts, bands of fibrous tissue can
form. This can cause adhesions that in effect bind the
contiguous organs together.

The most frequent symptoms that arise from endometriosis include: chronic pelvic pain, extremely painful
or crippling periods, pain during sex, painful bowel movements or discomfort in urination at the time of menstruation, and heavy bleeding, either with periods or between
them. The symptoms and their intensity vary greatly,
although between 60 percent and 80 percent of endometriosis patients do have some degree of pelvic pain.

The condition seems to worsen with time and as it
progresses may render a woman infertile. Women with
endometriosis who do conceive—and two thirds of those
who have the disease are able to—have an increased
rate of ectopic pregnancy and miscarriage. (The theoretical reasons for this are either that the prostaglandin
production from the implants impedes the movement of
the egg in the fallopian tube, or that the implants affect
the pelvic anatomy and interfere with the path of the
fertilized egg.)

The severity of symptoms does not always correspond with the relative advancement of disease. The smallest implants can induce as much pain as an extensive case of endometriosis.

Endometriosis is an incredibly common disease among women; it is estimated that five million women in the United States suffer from it. One reason it seems to be gaining in frequency is that women who delay childbearing are more likely to develop it. (Endometriosis rarely occurs in women before the age of twenty.) Another reason is that the disease has been difficult to diagnose. Laparoscopy, in regular use only since the 1970s, is considered the only certain way outside of major surgery to determine whether endometriosis has developed. Before laparoscopy, many women found themselves crippled with pain during their periods or during sex without knowing what was causing it.

It remains unclear what causes endometriosis. One theory, referred to as the "retrograde menstruation theory," is that during menstruation some of the endometrial tissue backs up in the fallopian tubes, emerges out the other side, and implants in the abdomen. Others contend that a lapse in the immune and/or hormonal system allows for endometrial growth outside of the uterus. Yet another theory is that the condition is genetic and the tendency to develop it is present from birth.

Endometriosis is not life-threatening, but it can be very wearing emotionally. In a full-blown case, it can interfere with a woman's job, sex life, and even social life. In sum, it can leave her feeling that she's lost control of her life. Women with endometriosis often find themselves on a seemingly endless quest for relief; some may begin to feel—or it is suggested to them— that their pain stems not from their pelvic region but from their imagination. It is a puzzling, infuriating disease, and because it's so misunderstood, having it can be lonely as well as painful.

HOW CAN A HYSTERECTOMY HELP?

Hysterectomy is about as close to a "cure" for endometriosis as there is. It's usually regarded as a last-ditch effort, to be undertaken after other treatments have been tried to no avail. For one thing, hysterectomy brings with it risks and repercussions that other treatments may not have. Also, it simply doesn't always do the trick.

One problem is that by the time hysterectomy is attempted, many of the implants are so entrenched that it could be difficult to remove them all. If the ovaries are left in place, the implants remaining behind may continue to respond as before, creating the persistent cycle of pain.

As for whether or not to take out the ovaries, one study found that if all the ovarian tissue is not removed, in 85 percent of cases the endometriosis will return. Others believe that if the ovary itself is not involved, there's no reason to extract it. It is often difficult, however, to determine the extent to which the ovaries are involved.

In addition, by undertaking hormone replacement therapy immediately after surgery, as many physicians would recommend, the endometriosis patient may well find herself right back where she started from. The Endometriosis Association recommends waiting at least three to six months before beginning estrogen replacement therapy. The sudden menopause may be difficult for a while, but that means the treatment is working and that the symptoms of endometriosis—which prompted the hysterectomy in the first place—are less likely to recur. Another approach, currently in the experimental stage, is to start hormone therapy a few months before the operation. This seems to allow the body to adjust to the hormone changes gradually while lowering the chances of the implants growing back.

Eileen was beginning to feel she was less a patient than a regular customer at the doctor's office. By age thirty-eight, she had been through a number of treatments for endometriosis, none of which eased her symptoms. She had a laparotomy to have the implants removed surgically, and a laparoscopy with laser; she was given Danocrine and Lupron. She felt horrible on Danocrine, and Lupron gave her side effects. And she was still in pain.

At this point Eileen decided she wanted a hysterectomy. She was married and had two stepchildren in their teens. She and her husband had their hands full with these two and were not planning to have any more. (He, in fact, had been considering having a vasectomy.) She was appalled, then, when her doctor—a new physi-

cian, since she had recently moved—suggested that she get pregnant instead.

To be fair, endometriosis does seem to regress upon pregnancy. So if a woman is planning to get pregnant anyway, she should be informed of this. But no one should have a baby to cure a disease. Eileen was sufficiently angry, however, to find another doctor, who ultimately performed the hysterectomy.

The sooner endometriosis is diagnosed, the better the chances that a nonsurgical treatment will suffice. Unfortunately, it's usually not caught until the disease has advanced to the point where nothing short of a hysterectomy could bring relief. We can hope that as more is learned about endometriosis and women and their doctors are better informed about which symptoms to look for, many more women will be able to catch up with their endometriosis before it overtakes them.

ALTERNATIVE TREATMENTS

As stated before, at this time there is no definitive, guaranteed treatment for endometriosis. It's more a matter of trial and error. Different women might respond better to one or another treatment depending on the progression of the disease, the location of the implants, and the severity and type of symptoms experienced.

Drug therapies

A number of hormone-based drug treatments are available. The theory behind this sort of treatment is to stop ovulation and menstruation in order to stall the bleeding and swelling of tissue that's triggered as ovulation and menstruation occur. What this actually does is create a false pregnancy or a false menopause. This is not a cure, but a way of easing the symptoms. Birth control pills, used on occasion in mild cases, can frequently keep such cases from getting worse. They usually cannot cure advanced cases. Before other drug therapies were available, they were often prescribed continuously instead of in the three-weeks-on, one-week-off cycle used for contraceptive purposes. Also, synthetic progesterone can be given either as a pill or injection to arrest the menstrual cycle completely.

One commonly prescribed medication is Danocrine, which is a testosterone derivative. There have also been promising results with the GnRH drugs described in Chapter 3, Fibroids.

Hormonal drug treatments should be tried before hysterectomy, but they are by no means perfect. All of them have side effects, some of which can prove difficult to tolerate. With Danocrine or GnRH analogs, menopausal symptoms are bound to occur, including vaginal dryness, hot flashes, and increased risk of osteoporosis. With Danocrine, weight gain, a decrease in breast size, nausea, leg cramps, hair growth, or a lower-pitched voice can occur. Some reactions will be temporary, but others may persist as long as the drug is taken. Aside from the sometimes prohibitive cost, another negative aspect of drug treatments is that once the drug is stopped, the endometriosis may recur.

Surgery

A number of surgical techniques besides hysterectomy can be used to reduce symptoms. One frequently effective approach is to cauterize or laser the growths through a laparoscope inserted in the abdomen. Recently, laser laparoscopies have been done so that the growths and adhesions are vaporized.

The advantage of such surgery is that you need to be in the hospital for only one day and that though several incisions may be required, they are all tiny. But it's important to realize that it's still *surgery* and that you stand a chance of needing a conventional surgical incision after all.

Performing this type of surgery, which involves bending down doing precise work for long periods of time, can be exhausting and arduous for a physician. Today it can often be done with videos, so the physician can watch exactly what's happening on the screen, which is much easier. The videotape can then go into the patient's records. This can prove helpful later on, if there are questions about fertility, for instance.

If the implants are found to be extensive, a laparotomy may be preferable to a laparoscopy. This is a more involved operation requiring a longer incision in the abdomen (usually a bikini incision or midline abdominal incision), and as a result, a longer period of recovery.

Again, the implants are cut, cauterized, or vaporized by a laser, cautery, or traditional surgical techniques.

Like the drug treatments, surgery for endometriosis is a way of buying time until the implants recede on their own. Both put the disease in a state of remission; the implants, and the pain that comes with them, could return. It may be several years before they do—if indeed they ever do—and these procedures can be repeated, although not indefinitely. The disadvantage to surgery is that additional adhesions can form, which in themselves can cause pain or compromise fertility.

Pain Control

Since the symptoms of endometriosis rather than the disease itself are the problem, merely treating those symptoms can keep it in check. Any effective form of pain management, then, may suffice.

Medication for pain is one obvious alternative. But here, the risk of addiction is a problem, particularly for women whose pain is severe. Some doctors sever the nerves that may be associated with pelvic pain by cutting the uterosacral ligament, which carries these nerves. This can be done through a laparoscope. One problem with this procedure is that women may experience a lessening of sensations during intercourse as a result. And studies have shown that significant pain relief occurs only in a small percentage of women.

But a great deal of research is being done on the management of pain, and you can discuss possible options with your doctor (see Chapter 6, Heavy Bleeding, Chronic Pain).

IS A HYSTERECTOMY A GOOD IDEA?

If you, like Eileen, find that your symptoms from endometriosis are intruding on your life and other methods
of controlling them have failed, a hysterectomy might
be advisable. Endometriosis is an unpredictable and
poorly understood disease, so if you have it, you should
become as informed about it as possible. Not all doctors
are well versed in the disease and its treatments, so you
should make the effort to find one who is. Because
endometriosis is a frequent cause of infertility, a fertility specialist might be a good candidate.

According to the Endometriosis Association, there
are unnecessary hysterectomies for endometriosis—but
not for the usual reasons. In this case, the operation
itself may be called for at the time that it's done.
Had the disease been detected earlier and appropriately treated, however, it might not have been needed
after all.

CHAPTER 6

Heavy Bleeding, Chronic Pain

Countless women are plagued by heavy bleeding during or between periods. Hysterectomy is one treatment for excessive bleeding, and about 10 percent of all hysterectomies are done for this purpose.

Bleeding problems generally fall into three basic categories. The first is heavy bleeding during regular periods. "Menorrhagia," as it is termed, can occur at any time in a woman's reproductive years. However, it is more likely to develop in the years approaching menopause. A woman who has enjoyed regular, trouble-free periods all her life and possibly has had children may suddenly find herself burdened by menstruation marked by heavy flows, if not outright gushes.

The bleeding can be severe enough to cause anemia or fatigue. But aside from the inconvenience and occasional stained clothing, it usually represents no serious health threat. This is not to underplay the life-disrupting capacity such bleeding can have, however; some who suffer from it may feel utterly paralyzed several days of each month. In rare cases it could be a sign of uterine cancer, and as always, heavy bleeding, and any other pathology, should be looked into.

Menorrhagia can often be attributed to small fibroids or polyps growing in the uterus. Another possible cause is a condition called "adenomyosis." Like endometriosis, endometrial tissue embeds itself in the myometrium, or the muscles of the uterus. As a result, the uterus becomes engorged and tender and there may be excess bleeding. Adenomyosis is often difficult to diagnose. The only sign may be a slight enlargement of the uterus.

Bleeding that crops up at odd times or lasts far longer than the normal period of menstrual flow is called "dysfunctional uterine bleeding." This often occurs when there is an "anovulatory cycle," which means that no ovulation takes place, and which can be the result of a hormone imbalance or a temporary effect of stress or illness. Another frequent cause of abnormal bleeding between cycles is benign cystic hyperplasia, in which an elevated estrogen level prompts an overgrowth of tissue in the endometrium. This is basically a benign condition, but it should be corrected because it can progress to more serious conditions. Untreated, it could develop into "adenomatous hyperplasia," the precancerous condition that could ultimately give rise to endometrial cancer. (Even some cases of hyperplasia, however, can be treated by methods other than hysterectomy.) Stress, too, can be a factor in both dysfunctional bleeding and menorrhagia.

Bleeding can also occur after menopause, either because of structural abnormalities, such as fibroids or polyps, or because of hormonal shifts. Anyone who starts bleeding six months or more after menopause should see her doctor to rule out cancer or precancerous changes.

CAN A HYSTERECTOMY HELP?

Hysterectomy can relieve heavy bleeding—if the cause of the bleeding is contained in the uterus. In many cases of heavy bleeding, however, the uterus is a perfectly healthy organ. It would be a shame to go through surgery and have a hysterectomy and then realize it could have been handled a far simpler way, such as by hormone treatments.

Every effort should be made to determine the cause of any excess bleeding. The bleeding itself is not the disease, but it may be a symptom of a number of gynecological or endocrine disorders. Bleeding might also be induced by certain prescription drugs or by another medical problem. It's important to be aware that heavy bleeding can also be the result of stress or emotional upset. Indeed, many cases of excessive bleeding elude clear diagnosis.

Another reason one should not leap into a hysterectomy is that *heavy bleeding* is a term so loosely defined it hardly means anything in itself. What one woman perceives as heavy bleeding may be viewed as moderate by someone else. If there is any question, a blood count may be done to see if the bleeding is causing anemia. Any *changes* in bleeding patterns should, of course, be noted, but even here normal fluctuations may occur. Bleeding itself has many connotations, and a woman who experiences unexpected bleeding understandably may be upset and concerned. But it's important to examine that bleeding in terms of the causes and possible effects on the woman's health.

Leanne had a number of episodes of heavy bleeding and went to her doctor, demanding a hysterectomy. The doctor felt this was not something to rush into, and did a D & C first. The uterus was normal but the bleeding continued. The doctor could see that her patient, visibly frustrated and upset, was determined to have definitive action taken. Since the doctor wasn't yet certain of the cause of the bleeding—which could have been aggravated by stress—she was reluctant to perform the operation despite her patient's pleadings. So she urged Leanne to seek a second opinion.

The consulting physician found that Leanne had an underactive thyroid. With thyroid replacement therapy her bleeding pattern returned to normal, and no hysterectomy was needed.

ALTERNATIVE TREATMENTS

D & C's are often recommended for women with heavy bleeding. Such a procedure can be effective if the cause of the bleeding is polyps or hyperplastic (overgrown) tissue and this tissue is removed. The operation might also be used diagnostically to determine that there is no cancer present to cause the bleeding symptoms. In this case, the results of the tissue examination may establish that a hysterectomy should or should not be scheduled.

The problem with D & C's is that any relief they provide may be temporary. The endometrium is scraped away during the procedure, but it immediately begins to grow back as the normal menstrual cycle is once again set in motion. If no treatable cause for the bleeding is found, such as a hormonal imbalance, the abnormal bleeding may recur. However, frequently the D & C offers several months or several years of more normal menstrual bleeding before the problem resurfaces.

One recently developed procedure with a number of advantages is a laser ablation of the endometrium. After a D & C has proven that no cancer is present in the uterine lining, the lining is actually destroyed with a laser. This is done through a hysteroscope, which is inserted through the cervix.

The operation requires only one day in the hospital and has a much lower risk of complication and side effects than hysterectomy. And since there is no incision, pain is greatly reduced. But as this is a new procedure and requires a specific laser, specialized equipment, and expertise in the technique, it is not yet widely available.

One drawback is that unlike some other options, a laser ablation of the endometrium is not for women desiring future children. A further consideration is that much is still not known about its long-term effectiveness. It's not clear, for instance, whether cancer could develop in any islands of endometrial tissue that remain. And, as with many new treatments, insurance companies may be reluctant to compensate for it.

A number of hormone therapies can effectively treat cases of heavy bleeding when a hormone imbalance is implicated. Oral contraceptives can moderate bleeding and may be prescribed for this purpose, if a woman is young, healthy, and a nonsmoker. Other possibilities are drugs mentioned previously, such as the GnRH analogs, Danocrine and progestins. As discussed in Chapters 3 and 5, hormonal treatments have a number of side effects that could be uncomfortable or raise the risk of other medical problems.

Depending on what triggered the bleeding, other treatments could be helpful. Any means of stress reduction, such as psychotherapy, meditation, or a program of exercise may, after a time, stem the blood flow. Correcting any vitamin deficiency or taking iron supplements for anemia may also be helpful.

Anyone who plans to have a hysterectomy because of heavy bleeding should do so only after very careful consideration. It is essential that all other options be thoroughly explored and that you be aware that the operation may not in fact be the best way to relieve the problem. To help rule out other potential causes of the bleeding, it's important to give your doctor as much information as possible about any patterns of the bleeding (for example, is it aggravated during times of stress?) and any other medications you may be taking.

PELVIC PAIN

Pelvic pain can take a number of forms. It can be a chronic, dull ache in the pelvic area; excruciating—nearly incapacitating—menstrual cramps; or pain during intercourse that virtually makes sex impossible.

CAN A HYSTERECTOMY HELP?

As with excessive bleeding, pelvic pain can be eased by hysterectomy, but only if the uterus is the source of the pain and no other cause can be established. Quite conceivably, someone in constant pain might feel desperate and be in a hurry to try anything that promises relief. The trouble is, there's no guarantee that hysterectomy will relieve the pain. Since it is major pelvic surgery, a hysterectomy could actually make pain worse. Also, the fact that such drastic action was taken to no avail could be devastating to someone who had invested so much hope in it. In cases where the pain has been psychologically derived, the point of pain may simply shift once the uterus is removed. Under such circumstances it would be far more effective to treat the *underlying* cause of the pain (through psychotherapy, etc.) rather than remove a uterus that bears no sign of disease.

Many women do have severe pain during their menstrual periods; and for some, it truly disrupts their lives. Sometimes it's a symptom of other problems, such as endometriosis, fibroids, or other tumors, and the pain can be treated by taking care of the primary cause.

Menstrual pain may occur by itself or along with other symptoms, such as headaches or nausea. Anyone considering a hysterectomy to relieve such problems should realize that the symptoms associated with the cramps (headaches, nausea, etc.) may not disappear with hysterectomy. It's also important to note that the severity of cramps may diminish with age and occasionally decreases after childbirth. If pain seems to intensify as time goes on, there may be other physiological factors that should be looked into.

The drug treatments for menstrual cramps available through prescription or over the counter contain anti-prostaglandins. These can irritate the stomach, and should not be taken on an empty stomach. Women with a history of ulcers should probably avoid this class of drugs. Oral contraceptive pills are also sometimes used to put severe menstrual cramps within the tolerable range. An interesting sidelight is that smoking appears to worsen menstrual pain, as nicotine has the effect of stimulating muscle activity in the uterus. So if you smoke, quitting can help ease your cramps (in addition to all the other benefits to your health).

Pain often has a psychological component. In some cases, it could be related to depression, for many people do express depression somatically. Pelvic pain could represent a displacement of emotional issues, such as conflicts about sex, femininity, or parenting. Psychological conditions like depression and stress can also lower a person's threshold of pain. Pain that has been perfectly manageable in the past may, in times of stress, suddenly seem unbearable.

There's often a reluctance to be open to emotional issues as a possible factor, because of the implication that the pain isn't *real*. But the pain *is* real, and any means of addressing that pain, whether it involves the body or the psyche, should be explored. Psychotherapy and other treatments for depression or stress might alleviate pelvic pain and could obviate the need for surgery altogether.

If the pain is of physical origin, every attempt should be made to diagnose the cause. Pain during intercourse could result from something as treatable as a vaginal infection, which can be detected during a routine pelvic exam. Such conditions as endometriosis or pelvic adhesions from previous operations could also underlie the problem, as could chronic pelvic congestion, which is when blood vessels in the pelvis dilate, obstructing blood flow (something like varicose veins in the pelvis). Depending on the severity of the problem, a hysterectomy may or may not be in order.

Another frequent cause of chronic or severe pelvic pain is pelvic inflammatory disease (PID). These infections can occur after childbirth or abortion, or, most commonly, when a sexually transmitted disease has been contracted. If you get a sexually transmitted disease while wearing an IUD, the chance of the complications may be increased.

The symptoms of PID include: pelvic pain (which occurs in about 18 percent of cases); fever; and a malodorous vaginal discharge. In most cases antibiotics can take care of the infection, but since the symptoms may be so slight as to be unnoticeable, they may not be caught early enough. This is particularly true of chlamydia, a PID now so widespread that any woman who is sexually active today should consider being tested for it.

Left untreated, PID can cause infertility or other reproductive problems, such as increasing the rate of ectopic pregnancy. In extreme cases, tubo-ovarian abscesses can develop. If they rupture, immediate surgery may be needed and sometimes that might mean a hysterectomy. It's important to note that having one episode of PID increases your vulnerability of getting another. Also, it's *always* essential to have any sex partner treated as well, for otherwise you risk becoming infected again.

There are ways to treat PID, short of hysterectomy. Antibiotics can be effective, even if the disease is advanced. Sometimes hospitalization is required, so large doses of antibiotics can be administered intravenously. If the disease has caused adhesions that have induced pain or compromised fertility, this can often be handled much the same way as endometriosis, with a laparoscopy or laparotomy. In many cases, fertility can be restored.

A hysterectomy should be done for pelvic pain only when every possible cause and potential alternative has been thoroughly explored. Your age, life-style, and other health conditions should be weighed into the decision as well. Because hysterectomy is no surefire cure for the problem, you really should have at least a second opinion before arranging for any major surgical intervention.

CHAPTER 7

Uterine Prolapse
and Sterilization

Uterine prolapse is when the pelvic floor—which is the shelf of muscle that props up the pelvic organs—starts to weaken and sag. In severe cases the uterus can drop into the vagina, and in *extreme* cases it can actually protrude down past the vaginal opening. Uterine prolapse is a condition rather than a disease, and unless other organs are affected, it is not dangerous. Perhaps 20 percent to 25 percent of hysterectomies are done because of a prolapsing uterus.

Prolapse usually occurs later in life, often after having many children—particularly after difficult births or births of large babies that strain the pelvic musculature. Genetic factors also contribute, with women in some families at an increased risk of prolapse. Chronic coughing (perhaps from smoking cigarettes or from asthma) can aggravate the problem.

The incidence of prolapse today seems to be declining, no doubt the result of improved obstetrical techniques, a trend toward smaller families, and better general fitness among women. A century ago this may well have been the most frequent "women's complaint" because of the conditions that existed then, including poor diet, hard physical labor imposed on many women, and, in a time when caesarean section was dangerous and not regularly performed, obstetric methods that sometimes left the pelvic area a shambles. Prolapse then was not only a common diagnosis but a popular one: doctors tended to blame misplaced uteri for nearly all women's health problems. It was called a "fallen womb," a term so close to "fallen woman" that it seemed almost to suggest some moral failing. Indeed, such things as tight lacing, sexual excess, and singing and dancing were thought to be its cause.

When the uterus prolapses, frequently other pelvic muscles have gone through a similar process of slipping and slackening. This condition in general is called "pelvic relaxation." There may be a rectocele, which is a hernia of the rectum that pushes into the back wall of the vagina. Someone with a rectocele may actually have to press on the bulge in the vagina in order to move her bowels. A cystocele is a hernia of the bladder into the vagina. As the bladder falls and the angle between the bladder and urethra changes, urinary leakage may result.

Other symptoms of pelvic relaxation include urinary difficulties, constipation, or lower abdominal pressure. Many who suffer from prolapse describe a sensation of heaviness, and some find sex to be unsatisfying if not positively uncomfortable. (That's because the vaginal muscles may have loosened and the uterus might have shifted position.)

A cystocele and rectocele may be surgically repaired without removing the uterus, but the prolapsing uterus may act as a weight and further threaten the support of any pelvic organs. If a cystocele and rectocele repair has been performed and the woman plans to have children, any subsequent deliveries should be by caesarean, as a vaginal delivery could weaken the tissues again. Serious prolapses tend not to occur until after a woman's childbearing years, so this is not often an issue. In most cases, the uterus is removed and the other organs are tacked up at the same time. Even this may not be a permanent cure. After hysterectomy and repair, the vagina may subsequently prolapse, and if repair is necessary, this may have to be done through an abdominal incision.

Uterine prolapse is most often detected during a pelvic exam, but if you've noticed any signs of it yourself, do call your doctor's attention to it.

ALTERNATIVE TREATMENTS

One option in the very early stages of uterine prolapse is to do absolutely nothing. If the descent is very gradual and produces no symptoms, you might not see any need to take action.

Probably a better choice at the initial phases would be to begin a program of exercise designed to tighten the muscles of the bladder, vagina, and rectum, muscles that might not be addressed in an ordinary workout. If you have trouble identifying these muscles, try while urinating to stop the flow of urine in midstream. Once you have isolated these muscles and can tighten them at will, do this in stages like an elevator ascent, stopping at five different levels as you progressively contract, then progressively relax the muscles. These exercises must be done daily for at least half an hour. Many women find that they are able to exercise while doing other things, such as washing dishes or watching TV. Although this routine doesn't really "undo" the slipping of muscles that has already begun, it may keep them from drooping further and can make the symptoms less noticeable.

Alisa began to notice the first signs of uterine prolapse a few years after her fourth child was born. She could feel some pressure on the bladder and had some loss of bladder control—symptoms similar to what she had in fact experienced during the last pregnancy. By the time she was forty-eight and started skipping periods, she was leaking a little urine whenever she coughed or sneezed.

At her doctor's suggestion, Alisa started doing exercises and made an effort to keep her bladder empty. She wears a mini-pad while exercising, but other than that she has no problem. She realizes that at some point she may need a hysterectomy, but for the time being she's just as happy to do without surgery.

Another alternative would be to take some form of estrogen replacement therapy. Because the dropping estrogen level of menopause is often a factor in the attenuating of muscles that causes prolapse, hormone replacement therapy can help prevent further deterioration. Whether this is an answer for you, however, depends on other factors that may or may not make hormonal treatments viable. This should be discussed with your doctor.

One further treatment is use of a pessary, a ring-shaped appliance made of rubber or plastic that fits in the vagina, something like a large diaphragm. Pessaries come in a variety of shapes and sizes to adjust for comfort and convenience. Most require that a doctor take them out, but others can be easily extracted, and some enable you to have sex without removing them. So if you have an active sex life—or any sex life, really—you should ask your doctor about one of these types. There are other devices that fill up the whole vagina, something like a plug. These would be appropriate only for someone for whom the ability to have sex is not an issue.

One disadvantage with the pessary is that it does need to be removed and cleaned periodically, approximately every three or four months. So depending on the type you have, this could mean a lot of trips to the doctor. And because it's a foreign material in your body, bacteria can collect, with odor, discharge, and irritation a possible result. For this reason women who wear pessaries have to take measures for extra hygiene, such as douching or antibiotic creams inserted into the vagina.

The pessary is often the best treatment for women in their seventies, eighties, and nineties, for whom surgery may be too physically taxing or may in fact be dangerous. Women with other health conditions that make them poor candidates for surgery (someone with heart disease or respiratory problems, for instance) should also seriously consider this option.

For the elderly woman who is not sexually active and not a candidate for extensive surgery, an operation to close off the vagina completely to keep the prolapsing organs in place may be considered.

STERILIZATION

There are women—more than a million a year, in fact—who seek hysterectomy as a way of insuring they won't have any more children. Technically, without a uterus a woman cannot give birth, so in that sense it is effective for birth control. But regarding other, less drastic measures that could be taken, that's where hysterectomy falls short. So much so that physicians have been urged not to perform hysterectomies for the intent of sterilization alone.

Contraception, remember, is of concern to a woman only until she reaches menopause. Hysterectomy means a permanent change in the body, a *series* of changes, really, of which the inability to conceive is only one aspect. There are a variety of options for birth control, each with its own advantages and drawbacks. Anyone who seriously, determinedly feels that nothing short of sterilization will suffice, tubal ligation (cutting and tying the fallopian tubes), which can be done on an outpatient basis, involves less than 10 percent of the risk of hysterectomy. Tubal ligation is a far less expensive form of treatment as well. When considering the cost of a procedure, you have to add in all the time lost from work or other activity *and* medical preparation and follow-up as well as the dollar amount a given operation costs.

In this country's medical community there has traditionally been a reluctance to perform hysterectomies for sterilization. A woman who wanted it done would somehow have to demonstrate that it was necessary. Sterilization has historically been associated with social control. In many cultures slaves or servants were intentionally castrated so they could not reproduce and would remain the subjugated class. There are people who regard unnecessary hysterectomies as discrimination against women, claiming that certain groups of women—minorities, the poor—are sometimes encouraged to have their uteri removed, often so they don't produce unwanted offspring. Today, a woman who *chooses* a hysterectomy for sterilization can probably find a doctor willing to perform it, but many doctors insist it is improper to perform a hysterectomy when there is no pathology to warrant it.

There are cases, however, where a hysterectomy could treat an underlying problem that could also be handled by less intrusive measures. If a condition like asymptomatic fibroids or mild uterine prolapse is present and the woman has planned to tie her tubes anyway, she might opt to schedule a hysterectomy. Many women are never quite comfortable with using birth control, sometimes because of religious considerations, sometimes because they never get to the point where they trust it. For them, news that they have, for instance, a mild uterine prolapse can actually seem a blessing in disguise: they can justify the hysterectomy and never again have to bother with contraception.

These situations have to be dealt with on a case-by-case basis. Hysterectomy is not a usual method of birth control—and it shouldn't be. Anyone leaning toward a hysterectomy because she wants to be sterilized should think it through very, very carefully. As discussed earlier, the uterus has functions other than those of childbirth and may have significance to the woman herself, significance she may not even be fully aware of until it's gone. The finality of the decision, too, may not come clear until that finality has hit. A definitive solution for birth control it is, but remember all that comes along with hysterectomy—the possible risks of surgery, effect on one's sex life, and hormonal changes as well.

CHAPTER 8

In the Hospital—and After

Whatever type of hysterectomy you have and whatever the cause, you need to prepare yourself for the reality that you are about to undergo a major operation. That hysterectomies are so common, and that some doctors may toss the term around as though it were nothing more serious than a tooth extraction, cannot take away from the fact that you *will* experience a substantial amount of discomfort and some pain, and that when all is said and done you will need a good chunk of recuperating time.

This latter point is especially true today, with insurance companies limiting the amount of hospital time they reimburse for. In the past a seven- to ten-day hospital stay was typical; today, if there are no complications, you might find yourself going home after four or five days.

Much of the apprehension before any operation stems from a fear of the unknown. Once you understand what is going to happen to you during those blurry hours in the operating room, you can go into the procedure with clearer expectations and greater confidence. Similarly, if you know ahead of time what kind of postoperative troubles you might run into down the line, you will be better able to deal with them. If you plan on running a marathon two days after you arrive home, you're going to be in for quite a shock—and quite a disappointment. If, on the other hand, you accept that there's a good chance you may be fatigued, you won't find the ensuing exhaustion as fierce a blow. Rather, you'll regard it as a temporary slowdown you'll have to pass through. And beyond that, you'll be able to arrange for extra help before-hand so you won't be doubly burdened with family or professional duties while trying to get back your strength.

Aside from information, the best preoperation prepa-ration you can give yourself is to make sure that when you go into surgery you're in the best overall health you can attain. The better physical condition you're in, the easier your recovery will be—and the lower the risk of complication. Maintain good nutrition, whittle away those extra pounds, get ample rest and exercise, and quit smoking once and for all. Not revolutionary advice, certainly, but important to keep in mind nonetheless.

Every woman's experience of hysterectomy will be different, depending on where and under what circum-stances she has it done, the state of her health, and how she feels about it, but there are certain events and ordeals most share.

You'll be admitted to the hospital either the morn-ing of the operation or the night before. At some point before the surgery you will probably have to fill out a medical history. It's important that you furnish as much information as you can here, even though it might not seem relevant to you at the time and despite the fact that you're about to be operated on and the last thing you want to do is answer a lot of questions. People respond differently to certain medications, for example, so noting down any adverse reactions you've had in the past would be helpful to your surgeon. Also, long-term health conditions your doctor may not yet be aware of may affect the course of treatment. The point is, you want to make it as unlikely as possible for a mistake or misunderstanding to occur.

You will also be required to sign a consent form, which grants your surgeon the authority to operate and the anesthesiologist the authority to administer anesthesia. While you may view this as a mere formality and write in your name without giving it a thought, the consent form should be taken seriously. Remember that it is your right to refuse treatment at any time if you wish and that you can state your priorities on the off chance that anything unexpected happens. If you want or need time to think about it, you can ask to see the form ahead of time. But under no circumstances should you feel forced to give a doctor carte blanche over your body.

As part of the hospital procedure, you will probably also have a thorough physical with a number of tests to insure your fitness for surgery, including blood tests, urine tests, a chest X ray, and an electrocardiogram. Your vital signs—meaning blood pressure, temperature, pulse, and respiration—will be checked periodically both before and after surgery.

In the weeks preceding the operation you may have donated up to three pints of your own blood in case the need for transfusion should arise at any point in surgery.

The hysterectomy operation is usually performed under general anesthesia, which insures that you will remain fully asleep through it. For patients who cannot have general anesthesia—those with severe cardiac or respiratory disease, for example, or those allergic to the anesthetic gas—a spinal anesthetic, which is local anesthetic injected in the area adjacent to the spine, is used instead. With a spinal or epidural anesthetic, the patient remains awake while the lower half of the body is numbed of pain. Surgery should take one to three hours, longer if there are any complicating factors.

Once out of the operating room you will be wheeled to the recovery room. After all indications confirm that your condition has stabilized, it's back to your hospital room. And for the next four to six days, this is pretty much where you'll be. For the first day you may have a catheter, a narrow tube inserted through the urethra and into the bladder, to monitor the output of urine, and eliminate the need to get up to go to the bathroom. You will also be given fluids intravenously for the first day or two after surgery, until your digestive system is able to handle fluids taken by mouth. Surgery and anesthesia tend to cause a temporary slowdown of bowel function. As bowel function returns, it's quite common to get gas pains. For some hysterectomy patients, in fact, this proves to be the most uncomfortable part of the whole experience.

Within a day or so of surgery you will be encouraged to walk and take deep breaths and cough to get your breathing and circulation up to par. Within three or four days you will probably be able to take light solid foods. Painkillers are usually given by injection for the first one or two days. After that, usually a mild pain pill will suffice. People vary in their tolerance for pain and need for pain medication. One patient, for example, had a long history of endometriosis and took virtually no medication after surgery. She said the postoperative pain was not as intense as what she had experienced every month with her menstrual period. On the other hand, if the pain relief is not sufficient, don't be afraid to ask for a stronger dose of medication.

It's important that you start taking an active part in your recovery when you're still in the hospital. Try to move about, sit up, and do minor exercises like moving fingers and toes, then work on your arms and legs. This helps to get your circulation going and avoid blood clots. As soon as the first day after the operation, you might try, with assistance, to walk. The catheter would probably be removed the day after surgery, so you will have to get up to go to the bathroom anyway. (In some cases when bladder repairs have been done the catheter may be kept in place much longer.)

As bowel function returns to normal the abdominal gas pains diminish and gas is passed rectally. This is a sign that you may begin to drink liquids and then start on solid food. Taking too much pain medication could delay the normal return to bowel function, so don't take any more than you need. You will probably move your bowels at least once before you leave the hospital.

You might get some additional symptoms when you get home. It's important to know what to anticipate so you'll have a sense of what should prompt a call to your physician and what you shouldn't be alarmed about.

One common symptom is to have some staining during the entire month or so after surgery. This has to do with the stitches dissolving at the top of the vagina. You may have to wear a pad as long as it lasts, but unless it's terribly heavy you needn't be concerned. If, however, a fever or vomiting occurs when you are home after the surgery, you should alert your doctor. Such a reaction could signal an infection or intestinal complication.

Similarly, you should consult a physician if you have severe pain. Any kind of pus or discharge at the site of the incision should also be checked. It's probably normal for there to be little scabs at the incision, but there's a chance the pus might suggest an infection. Many women have numbness or puffiness around the incision, but this should go away by itself after a couple of months. But whenever you have any symptoms and have any question about them, you should let your doctor know; the sooner any postoperative problem gets taken care of, the better.

Two days after she got home from the hospital, Karen was definitely not feeling well. She took her temperature, which was 100.5, and had vague abdominal cramping. None of this was horribly painful, but she made an office appointment with her doctor for the next day just to make sure everything was all right. The doctor did an examination along with a blood and urine test and it turned out she had a bladder infection. She got a prescription for antibiotics and felt better within a few days.

If you're employed, you can expect to stay out of work for four to six weeks. If most of your tasks are at home, it will probably take the same amount of time for you to feel completely up to them. There are huge individual variations with this, however. One woman may feel pretty well two weeks after surgery, with her strength gaining steadily and rapidly. Another may still feel quite fatigued six weeks postoperatively. There's no way to predict the pace of recovery. A smooth operation doesn't necessarily guarantee there will be smooth sailing from then on. If you feel you're dragging more than you thought you would be, check with your doctor. But it needn't suggest that there's anything wrong— nor does it imply you're going to be feeling that way forever.

What most women experience during this period is not pain but out-and-out exhaustion. You may feel the way you would when recovering from a horrible flu. This is not at all unique to hysterectomy, but true of any major operation. All your energy is going into the healing process. But hysterectomy is, for many women, their first experience with surgery and they may not be aware of the extent to which this can drain their resources. Also, many hysterectomy patients have felt perfectly well before surgery, so it can be frustrating to feel debilitated after.

The important thing is that you give in to your body's needs. Just as you can't play a 33 RPM record on 78, you can't try to put your body on a schedule it's simply not ready for. Sometimes the thought of responsibilities, the piling up of deadlines, bills, and laundry can lead someone to want to will herself into tiptop physical form. Many women feel they should always be doing things for other people and that it's wrong to put their own needs first. This is one instance where you have to give yourself priority—because by pushing yourself too far you may end up actually setting your recovery back. So rest, and take the time to let yourself get better.

Before the operation, you can take it upon yourself to minimize any difficulties you may face while recuperating. Women with small children should arrange for some assistance, for example. You may have to hire someone to help or enlist a neighbor or relative to ease your burden. You might consider preparing some meals ahead of time and putting them in the freezer so you won't have to bother later.

The point is that no one knows your particular situation but you. After the hysterectomy, your doctor is concerned with keeping you free of disease and physical complication. He or she won't know whether you have to navigate several flights of stairs to get in and out of your bedroom, need to drive several miles in order to buy a quart of milk, or have a number of employees depending on your judgment for everything they do. Knowing that you have things taken care of will greatly ease the stress you may confront when you face everyday life again.

As for how much you can do, you pretty much have to be the judge of that. People often ask whether it's okay for them to walk up and down the stairs. Use your own common sense. Try to take them slowly. Avoid climbing stairs too many times during a day. What you should clearly not do is any forced exercise and any physical activity that could strain the incision (such as heavy lifting). Also, because of the risk of infection, there should not be anything in the vagina for at least the first four weeks. That means no intercourse, no using tampons, and no swimming. A shower would be preferable to a tub bath during this time.

While people do recover at different rates, be aware of the typical time frame. If you feel after a week that you want to go to work, think twice about it.

Thirty-four-year-old Jeannine ran her own public relations firm. Her business was beginning to pick up a number of accounts when a diagnosis of adenomatous hyperplasia required that she have a hysterectomy. She had been on hormonal treatment for this, which was not successful in reversing the condition. Aside from abnormal bleeding, she hadn't felt ill before the operation, but she felt great in the hospital and terrific when she got out. The first day home, someone called from the office about a mix-up with one of her clients, so she decided to come into work to straighten it out herself.

She came in the next couple of days to follow up on the project, but when morning arrived on the fourth day, she couldn't even get out of bed. She was alarmed when she could hardly move all day, and arranged to see her doctor later in the week. There were no complications; she had merely pushed her body too far. She realized she could not just jump into the middle of a stressful routine and so she compromised: for a while she would have some important work sent home to her. This way she felt in touch with what was happening at work, without having to go full force.

In many ways your return home is not the end of the recovery period, but rather the beginning of another phase of it. You will be tired; you may still have pain (though it is unlikely you will require any prescription pain medication); and you're likely to encounter some vaginal discharge or light bleeding. (Anything that seems unusual, such as heavy bleeding or clotting, smelly or heavy discharge, fever, or severe pain, could signal an infection or other complication and should be reported to your physician.) It will undoubtedly take some time before you can resume your daily activities without experiencing some degree of discomfort or all-out exhaustion. This could go on for a few weeks or it could take longer. The more assistance you have previously arranged to accommodate this, the better.

Recovery means not just that the stitches have been removed and the pain subsides; it is above all a period of healing that involves both body and mind. You have to adjust to your body after the operation, and the

changes and stresses you've been through may well
have taken their toll. Many women do feel teary or
depressed at some point. For some it could occur during the hospital stay, often when the concern about the
operation itself has passed and the woman is forced to
confront her own feelings about hysterectomy. With
others it creeps up on them weeks or even months
afterward.

---

*After her hysterectomy for endometrial cancer, An-
nette, a forty-five-year-old lawyer, leapt right back into
her life. There was no sign of spread, no complication
in surgery. She started working part-time barely a week
after she had left the hospital and soon her schedule
and pace were back to normal.*

*Then about six months after the operation an elderly
aunt passed away. Suddenly, Annette fell apart. She felt
extremely depressed and exhausted. Her relative's death
apparently triggered her own feelings and fears about
death. Before and immediately after the hysterectomy,
she hadn't dealt with the fact of having cancer. Instead,
she had put all her energy into her career, using her
job as an excuse not to confront these painful feelings.*

*Annette took a restful vacation and went to see a
therapist a few times. Ultimately she did give herself a
chance to fully absorb emotionally what it was she had
faced.*

Feelings that seem prompted by hysterectomy are
not something you should deny to yourself or to any-

body else. Having them does not mean that you're emotionally unstable and certainly doesn't imply that you're crazy (even though many doctors fail to acknowledge that some type of emotional swaying is more than likely to occur). This is a natural part of the process and you need to *go* through it in order to *get* through it. Some women report that an entire year had to pass before they felt truly themselves again.

However long it takes you, it is helpful at this point to have some support in your life. An open and supportive relationship with a spouse, good friends, psychological counseling, or a support group can do wonders to smooth things through. It's up to you to approach those who can support you, and regardless of who else is in the picture, to treat yourself well. If any depression goes on too long or gets too severe, however, you may be wise to seek professional help (see Chapter 10).

The physical side of recuperation does need to run its course. If, however, several months go by and you still don't feel yourself, you probably should check with your doctor. A protracted recovery could signal other problems resulting from the surgery, such as anemia, infection, or a hormone imbalance.

The period during which you're rebuilding your strength could also be a good time to build new health—to start improved health habits and abandon poor ones. Many women, for example, quit smoking when they're in the hospital. It's already discouraged since they can't smoke in the room, and any breathing trouble they have can make them aware of the damage each puff could be doing to their bodies. You can reevaluate your dietary habits. Many things creep into our diets that aren't good for us. You don't need to completely overhaul your life-style. Small changes can be helpful, for instance, switching from boxed cereal to oat bran or from fast food to meals that feature fresh fruits and vegetables.

And recovery, a time when you can't exercise, may in fact be just the time to think about your own fitness program for when you're finally up and about. Being temporarily down and tired can make you appreciate good health more than ever before. Also, for many women hysterectomy prompts fears about aging. Exercise keeps you feeling young—aside from all its other health benefits—so what could be a better antidote?

Throughout the process of hysterectomy, you've undoubtedly learned a great deal about your body. This new awareness can have very positive results: you'll know more about what your body needs; you'll be better able to detect any changes that could require medical attention; and you'll have a new understanding of the importance of doing things for your health.

CHAPTER 9

Risks and Complications

As with any operation, when you decide to have a hysterectomy you're subjecting yourself to some degree of risk. It's true that most women do emerge from their surgery—given the appropriate recovery time—healthy and feeling as well or better than they did before. Yet there are instances where, because of complications, additional surgery is needed or other physical problems arise that leave them feeling worse. It's worth pointing out that the more serious the condition that led to the hysterectomy, the more likely are complications to occur.

According to research, between one quarter and one half of all women who undergo hysterectomies will suffer some complication. Most of these are minor, and very short-lived. However, it's essential that you remain aware of this as you make your decision—particularly since the risk associated with many of the nonsurgical alternatives is much lower.

The first risk to note is that presented by the mortality rate, the risk of death. This rate turns out to be between one and two deaths for every thousand hysterectomies performed. The risk of dying as a result of a hysterectomy is lower than that of many other types of surgery, but it's still a greater risk than you may face with other less invasive procedures—including, in many cases, doing nothing.

These improbable cases of death may be the consequence of rare complications arising during the operation (severe infection, blood clots in the lung or brain, extreme reaction to anesthesia) or of conditions that existed previously (such as cardiac or pulmonary disease). The risk of death is highest in hysterectomies related either to pregnancy or to cancer, which are those most likely to be done on an emergency basis. This is not to start you worrying, however. Under no circumstances are the odds against you.

Here is a list of the most common types of complications following hysterectomy, arranged roughly in their order of prevalence. These situations will occur in a small number of women. They are not totally preventable. You can minimize the chances by having a highly skilled and experienced physician, but you can never say for sure that such complications won't happen.

1. *Fever.* By far the most frequent complication is postoperative fever. The cause is frequently a bladder infection (often related to the catheter), or an infection at the operative site. The incidence of fever is slightly higher with a vaginal hysterectomy.

This is generally treated, quite effectively, with antibiotics. With a vaginal hysterectomy, many physicians will prescribe antibiotics at the time of surgery as a preventive measure. This may reduce the chance of developing fever, diminish the need for subsequent medication, and shorten the length of the hospital stay. In the case of abdominal hysterectomies, the effectiveness of preventive antibiotics is less clear.

2. *Postoperative atelectasis*. This is the effect of your lungs not expanding fully in the period after surgery. This results in part from the effect of the anesthetic, and in part because deep breathing may cause abdominal pain after surgery and you may take shallow breaths to avoid the discomfort.

The way to handle this is to force yourself to cough and take deep breaths as soon as possible after surgery. The nurses on the staff should be able to help you. Many women are reluctant to do this, fearing that the incision will open up if they cough. First, assure yourself that this will not happen, and second, try holding a pillow or towel against your abdomen. This may prove more comfortable for you. It's important that you work on breathing during the first day or two after surgery, even if it hurts at first. The more you do it, the faster that discomfort will fade.

Some people, often those who have chronic respiratory problems, may need additional help, perhaps an oxygen mask with built-in pressure.

One way you can guard against this problem is to be in good general health . . . and not to smoke. It's also advisable to look into changing your date of surgery if you develop a bad cold or respiratory ailment as you approach the time of the operation.

3. *Urinary difficulties.* There is a wide range of bladder problems that can occur. As already mentioned, the most common is a simple bladder infection, which is easily treatable.

Then there's the possibility of the bladder becoming overdistended after surgery. This may occur if the catheter has not been used or has been removed before you are alert enough to know when your bladder is full. This may interfere with the bladder-emptying mechanism and may make it difficult to control. If this occurs, a catheter may have to be inserted and left in place for a few days. After the catheter is removed, it's important to try to urinate frequently on your own to avoid a recurrence of this problem. Also, alert someone on the medical staff to any burning, urgency, or other discomfort so a culture can be taken.

4. *Bowel difficulties.* Temporary paralysis of the bowel after a hysterectomy is a quite common complaint, most frequently with an abdominal hysterectomy and when there have been pelvic adhesions.

A sluggish bowel may cause cramps or bloating that, though uncomfortable, are not serious. The reasons for the condition could be the fact of not having eaten, the relaxing effect of the anesthetic or subsequent painkillers, the effect of surgery or the digestive disorientation that often comes with being in a strange place or eating according to a different schedule.

In a certain percentage of women there is quite a long delay before the bowels start operating again, and their distended bellies may attest to that. All that's usually done is to keep the patient from eating solid foods for a few days, or to put a tube down the gastrointestinal tract to remove any gas.

As a preventive measure, you could discuss this with your doctor ahead of time. Some women benefit from being on a liquid or low-residue diet for several days in advance of surgery.

5. *Anesthetic complications.* In the old days severe nausea and vomiting were common reactions to anesthesia. Acute allergic responses can affect the heart and lungs. Today the knowledge of anesthesia and methods of applying it have made this quite unlikely. Some people are going to have some reaction no matter what. If you've ever had complications from anesthesia before, be sure to tell your doctor.

In some rare situations, people lack an enzyme to metabolize the anesthetic. They may not wake up for several days and will need to be on a respirator until the time they do. As this enzyme deficiency tends to run in families, inform your doctor beforehand if this has ever happened to a relative of yours.

With anesthesia, however, it's important to realize that no one is simply going to hook you up to an IV and knock you out. Before any anesthesia is given, you will have submitted a detailed medical history, and will have talked with an anesthesiologist or nurse anesthetist. If you have any fears about the anesthetic—and for many the notion of being "out" and not in control can be frightening in itself, especially if they've never been under an anesthetic before—raise them with a professional. Your questions should be answered and any fears allayed.

Andrea was quite nervous about taking anesthesia for her hysterectomy—more nervous, in fact, than about the surgery itself. Although her asthma usually stayed under control, she had had a couple of attacks that landed her in the emergency room. If anything happened during the operation, she wondered, what could she do?

She discussed this with her doctor, and they settled on using a spinal anesthetic. The doctor explained that she might feel some sensation during the procedure—tugging and pressure, perhaps. And if she should get too uncomfortable, she could be given sedation, in the form of intravenous valium, as well. Thus assured, Andrea had the hysterectomy without complications.

---

6. *Blood loss*. In general, more than one in ten hysterectomy patients will require a blood transfusion. This percentage may be artificially high, however, because the need for transfusion often stems from preexisting health conditions, such as anemia. If you start out with a good blood count, your chances of having a transfusion will be less. If you do lose some blood, you might need no more than iron pills after surgery.

The possible need for a transfusion is much greater with myomectomies than with hysterectomies (see Chapter 3, Fibroids). Certain other situations raise the incidence of transfusion, such as pelvic infections, previous pelvic surgery, pelvic scar tissue, or extensive endometriosis. You can check with your doctor to see if a transfusion is anticipated and discuss any options you might have in preparing for this.

Today all blood used for transfusions is tested for every known disease, including hepatitis and AIDS. The chief concern is that there may be diseases we just don't know about yet, or that the disease is present at such an early stage that it cannot yet be detected. For example, if someone contracts the AIDS virus, it may be several months before the blood test is positive.

Because of concern, some women choose to donate their own blood on the off chance that it may be needed. If so, this should be done the month before surgery—it cannot be done just the day before the operation, as you need some time to build up your blood count after the donation. Some hospitals allow someone you know, perhaps a spouse or family member, to donate blood for this purpose. This practice is controversial, though, because their blood can't be assumed to be safer than anyone else's and must be tested as vigorously as any other blood.

7. *Injury to the urinary tract*. Injury to the ureter, the tube that runs from the kidney to the bladder, occurs in two to five cases for every thousand hysterectomies; the rate for bladder laceration (tearing) is be-

tween three and eight cases per thousand. These organs are vulnerable because they lie quite close to the uterus. The ureter is most likely to sustain injury either high up near the ovary or at the point where it's next to the cervix, as it passes by both.

In a radical hysterectomy, the sensory nerves of the bladder are prone to be cut. This could interfere with one's sensing the need to urinate and with controlling bladder function. Another common, minor injury is that the bladder may be slightly bruised while being dissected from the uterus. This can cause difficulty urinating, but the use of a catheter for short time should take care of it.

Monitoring the placement of these organs can lessen the chance of injury, and prompt recognition and repair can minimize ensuing complications. It's best for tears to be sewn up right there on the operating table. Such repairs might prolong recuperation time but should not lead to any long-term complications. If injuries are not discovered until later, when symptoms start to give clues as to their whereabouts, the treatment is a bit more complex and needs to be dealt with on an individual basis.

In most cases these injuries can be seen, but with cancer, extensive endometriosis, or severe infection the view may be obstructed. A bladder injury can be especially difficult to detect because the edge of the bladder is not always easily distinguishable from the surrounding tissue. There have been occasions when a stitch has been inadvertently placed in the bladder. As a result, after the operation urine may begin to flow through the top of the vagina and out. This is termed a "fistula," and once recognized, this, too, may be repaired, but then may require subsequent surgery.

8. *Injury to the intestine*. Either the small or large intestine could be injured when the abdominal wall is opened during surgery or if one or both of the organs is abnormally stuck to the abdominal wall. There may be adhesions attaching the bowel (large intestine) to the uterus, possibly at the cervix.

Again, if any injury sustained is quickly caught, it can usually be sewn up then and there with little further difficulty. However, the patient may have to have a temporary colostomy. This is a drainage of excretory contents through the abdominal wall to allow for the affected area to heal. The temporary colostomy would be removed in a second operation a month or two later.

Another problem is that scar tissue can develop in the abdomen after surgery, possibly causing pelvic pain or digestive difficulties. About 2 percent of hysterectomy patients will need further surgery to remove such scar tissue from the bowel.

9. *Clotting*. A thrombosis, or blood clot, that could develop as a complication of surgery may threaten to block off a blood vessel partially or completely. It is most likely to develop after a period of immobility (a time when your blood flow can grow sluggish). Those at the highest risk of having a dangerous clot include women who smoke, are overweight, or take pills with a

substantial estrogen content, such as birth control pills or estrogen replacement therapy.

A clot tends to form in the lower half of the body but may travel to the lungs (where it is termed a pulmonary embolism). Early signs to watch for are swellings in the leg or ankle, soreness on movement, or tenderness midcalf. If the problem occurs in the lungs, you might get pain when you breathe, or a dry cough. If the clot has developed in abdominal blood vessels, the earliest sign may be when it travels to the lung.

Let your physician know if you have any of these symptoms. This is a serious, potentially life-threatening complication. Clots can usually be treated with anticoagulant medication, but occasionally more extensive treatment may be needed.

10. *Residual ovary syndrome.* Pain during sex may occur when the ovaries have been left in. Before a hysterectomy, the uterus is at the top of the vagina, the ovaries at the sides. With the uterus gone, the ovaries tend to be pulled in, and frequently rest at the top of the vagina. Sometimes they can adhere to the vagina. The ovaries are quite sensitive (like a man's testicles), and if they're placed toward the center, there can be some discomfort. (This can happen when the uterus is in place, although a hysterectomy makes it more likely.) When pain occurs during intercourse, try to avoid positions where there's penetration in that particular area. If pain persists, do see your physician to check for other possible causes.

CHAPTER 10

Weight Gain, Depression, and Other Aftereffects: Real or Imaginary?

A long list of symptoms has been linked to hysterectomy. Some of these can be explained by hormonal changes, some by the operation itself, and still others may be coincidental. Many women are concerned about the possible aftereffects of surgery, and it may help to clarify what these may be . . . as well as suggest remedies for them.

The first point to make is that no side effect is universal. Depression, for example, is not an inevitable consequence of hysterectomy even though many women who have hysterectomies do suffer from depression to some degree. Many side effects that arise after the operation are, in fact, linked to other conditions that affect your health (age, level of fitness, nutritional habits, etc.). Certain aftereffects can be minimized or even avoided altogether by preoperative preparation (counseling, quitting smoking, etc.). In most instances, you should be able to control symptoms and maintain good health, either by taking the proper hormonal therapies or by altering your own health regimen. One more thing—any symptom that you experience is not imaginary. Whatever you feel is *what you feel* and should be regarded as a valid health issue.

1. *Weight gain.* This is listed first not because it's the most common, but because it's among women's chief concerns about the operation. Some women do seem to put on some pounds after a hysterectomy, but this is probably due to factors other than the surgery itself.

Women most frequently undergo hysterectomies between the ages of forty and sixty. This is also the time when they—menopausal or not—tend to run into weight problems. Women who may have scoffed at the idea of dieting in their twenties and thirties now find themselves battling against unwanted pounds, especially those that stubbornly settle around the hips and abdomen. This occurs at least in part because metabolism slows down at about this stage of life, so the body burns calories at a slower rate. A woman who has had a hysterectomy may attribute her weight gain to the operation, although it is bound to have occurred anyway.

In addition, the recovery period may keep a woman off her feet for a while, longer if she has any complications. At a reduced level of exercise the metabolism lopes along at a sluggish pace, so if she doesn't lower her caloric intake accordingly, she'll inevitably put on weight. Without exercise the muscles start to slacken and turn flabby, so even if a woman doesn't actually gain weight, she may indeed feel fatter.

Another possibility is, quite simply, that some women may load on calories in the weeks or months following a hysterectomy. People eat—and overeat—for various reasons. Many people turn to stuffing themselves when they're depressed, and depression can at times follow hysterectomy. Similarly, there are those who overdose on food when their self-image lags. This is, of course, counterproductive because after the initial gratification the food brings, they're only going to feel worse.

The process of recovering from an operation might itself lead many to overeat. After a period of fasting, sometimes your appetite returns with a vengeance. Hearty eating then becomes connected in your mind with feeling better, and you could acquire the habit. In other instances, you may be lying around feeling sorry for yourself because you're bedridden and bored. Eating, then, might merely be something to do. Or you might be completely drained of energy and assume that more food is going to give you more punch. True, you do need to eat, but overeating will only add fat—not vigor. If you feel utterly lacking in energy, it might be advisable to take a multivitamin or, if you've lost much blood, an iron pill.

If the prospect of gaining weight concerns you, talk to your doctor or a nutritionist. Someone who is prone to overweight or overeating may benefit from following a structured diet for the initial months after the operation. Anyone who has a balanced, healthy, not-too-caloric diet and makes an effort to exercise should not have to worry about extra pounds creeping up when she's not looking. Since a hysterectomy does represent a break in routine, it can be a good time to reevaluate your regular diet and make sure it's a good one. Emphasize quality in foods, not quantity, address any underlying reasons for overeating, and there will be no need for you to be plagued by excess weight.

2. *Depression*. Depression after hysterectomy is a complex matter because there are so many possible sources of depression. Hormonal changes can easily prompt depression, and thus a woman may well be afflicted by mood shifts after a hysterectomy. Depression may hit someone at any time of hormonal fluctuation: adolescence, pregnancy, starting or stopping birth control pills, menopause, and, for many, every single month. It seems that some are more susceptible to this than others; thin people often feel it more, whereas heavy people tend to notice it less. (Perhaps because some hormones are stored in their fat.) When the hormone changes are abrupt—as they are with hysterectomy, especially when the ovaries are removed in premenopausal women—it may strike with greater severity.

Remember that once your body gets attuned to the new level of hormones, your moods are likely to even out; women who fall into depression during menopause are not depressed their whole lives. Hormonal therapies can soften the effects, but this is not always an option for everybody (see Chapter 11). If not, there are alternatives, such as counseling, group therapy, or other medication.

Or you can just decide to stick it out. Women who go through menopause and don't take hormones may have some changes in mood and sex drive; but once they adjust naturally, they can have a greater strength afterward.

Interestingly, in cultures where old age is revered and women in their postmenopausal years are granted high status, women are not bothered by menopausal depression and other symptoms. This suggests that there may in fact be a sociological element to this depression. In our youth-crazed culture, signs of aging—even the sighting of a few wrinkles—can make a woman feel less attractive, less worthy as a person, and ultimately, depressed.

Pauline, an anthropologist who had studied the role of women in many societies, decided that she was not going to let her own culture dictate what happened to her body—and how she'd feel about it. She said she "wasn't interested in trying to be young" and chose not to take hormone therapy after she had a hysterectomy at age forty-eight. She uses a lubricant when she has sex, but other than that she has sensed little change.

Attitude is important. Women who are willing to accept mild depression and other hormonal changes are generally not terribly troubled by it. Women who had been set on taking hormones tend to be more affected by depression. In the following case, the hormonal effects coupled with an ambivalence about aging that had been stirred up by the hysterectomy left the woman nearly devastated emotionally.

An actress who had a hysterectomy at age forty-six, Barbara was not a candidate for hormone therapy because she had been diagnosed as having endometrial cancer. This came as a shock to her and she was severely depressed. She was concerned about her sex life and nearly frantic about her career—quite attractive, she had long been able to compete with much younger women. She feared that not being able to take hormones to keep her skin smooth was going to put her over the very edge she had been hovering on for a long time.

Ultimately, she accepted the fact that she was not going to be an ingenue forever, and found herself playing other roles. Although it disturbed her for a while, she was able to accept the fact that she couldn't postpone her aging and took it in stride.

Aside from hormonal changes, there are a number of reasons depression could strike a woman emerging from a hysterectomy. As discussed in Chapter 1, the awareness of her capacity to give birth often plays an important part in a woman's self-concept. What may be equally important is that others view her this way. So if a woman feels part of her role is to have children and now suddenly she can't, she may have a crisis of identity and grow depressed. Perhaps as our culture comes to regard women as other than baby-producing machines, depression might prove less of a factor.

With emotional issues, it's important to remember we're dealing on both conscious and unconscious levels. A woman may consciously be glad she no longer has to worry about birth control, while unconsciously she's mourning the loss of her childbearing ability. These unconscious feelings may never get articulated, not even to herself, but she may become depressed as she fails to resolve them. Similarly, a woman may be consciously grateful to her physician for relieving the problems she had before the hysterectomy, but somewhere underneath she's angry with the doctor for depriving her of her uterus.

Because we've often grown up feeling that it's not appropriately feminine behavior to express anger, it's common for women to repress such emotions. Such supressed feelings are sometimes turned inward and experienced as depression. For many women depression may represent a displacement of other feelings or conditions. For example, some women respond to stress by becoming depressed. Since a hysterectomy can be stressful on many levels—physical and otherwise—it could thus be a source of depression. A depressed state can also result from a woman's feeling she lacks control. And many women do feel they lack control over their bodies and their lives when they go through surgery or even through menopause; all these things just happen to you, even *overwhelm* you, and you might feel helpless as a result.

There have been a number of studies on post-hysterectomy depression. Their conclusions as to the percentage of women who get depressed vary (some say about a third; some, half; some, less), but they do point to certain patterns. Some research has concluded that many women react to hysterectomy according to the "stress response syndrome," which is a symptomatic response to traumatic life events. This is generally characterized by the intrusion of unpleasant thoughts and attempts to fend off painful memories and feelings. When the trauma inherent in a given situation—such as the death of a loved one, a divorce, or major surgery—is not sufficiently worked through, there can be a "numbing" of related feelings as the emotional conflicts continue to stir, though perhaps unconsciously.

The path of post-hysterectomy emotions described in the study by Kaltreider in the *Journal of the American Medical Association* is reminiscent of that associated with any great personal loss, with denial and anger ultimately wending their way toward acceptance.

1. *Outcry:* "Oh, no, it can't be true."
2. *Denial:* "Nothing has changed."
3. *Intrusiveness:* "I am defective and unlovable."
4. *Working through:* "I am changed but am still myself."
5. *Completion:* "I will go on with my life."

What transpires is that many of the negative and fearful feelings are initially held back by hysterectomy patients. In the period during and immediately after surgery, many women express a "determined cheerfulness." According to one report, 78 percent conceded that they had hidden feelings of fear (about mortality, changes in sexuality, etc.) from their male doctors. Between six weeks and six months later, such women were often beset with spells of anxiety and melancholy. The swings in mood sometimes persisted for well over a year.

A woman's depression often comes as a surprise to family members who had taken pride in what a good sport she has been through it all. Frequently—because by that time the hysterectomy is thought to be history—the woman fails to make the connection between the operation and her state of mind. As a result, she may not know to seek the appropriate counseling.

Another study found that women who underwent emergency hysterectomies experienced a greater threat to their self-concept than those who had some time to adjust to their impending surgery. This suggests that a period of reconciliation or "mourning" is essential, and that if the opportunity doesn't present itself before surgery, it will have to be caught up on later.

All this points to the importance of addressing the emotions prompted by hysterectomy whenever they might arise. Since the emotional wounds often crop up well after the surgical wounds have healed, you may no longer be in regular contact with the doctor who operated. And the doctors who focus on the organic complaint may not be as vividly aware of the emotional aftereffects of surgery and thus not think to prepare you for the possibility. Do what you can to deal with your feelings before the operation. If you're not comfortable discussing them with your doctor, find another professional you can talk to.

Certain women appear to be more prone to post-hysterectomy depression. Women under forty, especially those who had hoped to have more children, may be hit exceedingly hard, for instance. Women who have had no clear symptoms of pathology leading to the operation tend to feel it worse than those for whom hysterectomy represents a definite curative measure. Women with a history of depression as well as women lacking social support (family, friends, community, support groups, etc.) are also more likely to succumb to emotional lows.

Much of it comes down to how the woman herself has perceived the operation. If she sees it as something she had little control over, something done *to* her, she could well sink into a depression. If, on the other hand, she regards the surgery as a positive way of addressing her own health needs—as an action that could liberate her from pain and future medical problems—then it may not rattle her emotionally.

3. *Hysterectomy and the healthy heart*. Because of the many physical changes that go hand in hand with hysterectomy, there are other possible long-range effects on your health. The human body is more than an assemblage of individual organs; all its parts work together, and when there's a change in one area, other systems are likely to be altered as well.

Research indicates that hysterectomy is associated with an increased risk of heart disease. This is of concern because cardiovascular disease is the leading cause of death in this country. Early in life, women have a lower rate of cardiovascular disease than men, but after the age of sixty the sexes are pretty much even. Around menopause women become increasingly susceptible to cardiovascular ailments, primarily because estrogens play a protective role. A surgical menopause seems to push the rate up even faster. Some studies have suggested that following a hysterectomy, premenopausal women face a threefold increase in coronary heart disease.

When we talk of cardiovascular disease, we're generally referring to two forms: coronary artery disease, where fats build up in the arteries and can cause an obstruction in circulation; and hypertension (high blood pressure). Often both are present. Coronary artery disease can lead to heart attacks, atherosclerosis, and severe chest pain (angina pectoris). Hypertension increases the risk of heart attack and can cause stroke.

The precise effects of hysterectomy on cardiovascular health are not clear. Cholesterol does seem to accumulate in the arteries faster without the presence of the ovaries. Removing the ovaries, particularly in younger women, seems to provoke the steepest rise in the incidence of cardiovascular disease, but taking out just the uterus appears to make a difference as well. This indicates that the uterus may offer protection—or that somehow it contributes to the protection the ovaries provide. It's also conceivable that the operation itself may cause sufficient stress to compromise cardiovascular health.

The cardiovascular system is affected by both physiological and life-style factors. Many people are naturally prone to certain conditions, such as high blood pressure. A tendency toward particular problems seems to run in families. Those who feel they are at risk of cardiovascular disease can take some preventative measures. It's important to monitor how you're feeling and to bring any changes (chest pains, numbness, palpitations) to the attention of your physician. Also, you should have routine cholesterol and blood pressure checks.

In addition, you can eliminate factors that could have set your cardiovascular health on the wrong path. One place to start is with nutrition. It's essential to maintain a good, nutritionally balanced diet, keeping the fat content low. Use moderate amounts of salt. (Excess salt can raise blood pressure among certain people. As a nation, we probably oversalt our food anyway, so it can't hurt to cut back a bit.) Obesity can be a strain on the heart, so whittle away those excess pounds. If you're severely overweight or have other health problems, it's probably best to lose weight under a doctor's supervision. If you're diabetic, you should maintain blood sugar levels within the appropriate range.

Moderate exercise also brings many benefits to cardiovascular health. Aerobic exercises enhance your intake of oxygen and minimize the accumulation of cholesterol—to say nothing of keeping all of your musculature in shape and making you *feel* better in general. Don't fall into the habit of being sedentary.

Stress puts a good deal of wear and tear on the cardiovascular system. A certain amount of stress is unavoidable in today's world, but sometimes we let it take us over and allow minor mishaps and annoyances to get blown out of proportion. Learning to manage stress is essential to maintain good health. Exercise, meditation, therapy, and relaxation training are but a few ways to cope with stress in your life. You should explore to find which means work for you.

Quitting smoking is probably the one best single action you can take to lower your risk of heart problems. Smoking raises blood pressure and speeds up the heart rate while limiting the absorption of oxygen into the bloodstream. It also promotes the accumulation of fat in the arteries, which can result in atherosclerosis, heart attacks, strokes, and other circulatory diseases. Cardiovascular disease, not lung cancer, is thought to be the leading cause of death among smokers. Any way you look at it, smoking is bad news for cardiovascular health—but the good news is that you can quit.

4. *Guarding against bone loss.* Having a hysterectomy and removal of ovaries puts women at a greater risk of developing osteoporosis—the loss of calcium that leaves bones porous and brittle, and thus vulnerable to fracture. It is quite common among postmenopausal women. About one fourth of all women over age sixty are afflicted by it to some degree, and fully half of women whose menopause is surgically induced suffer from it as well. After menopause, women lose bone at twice the rate of men, most of it occurring in the first few years that follow. Like many conditions, there seems to be a tendency for it to run in families.

After a hysterectomy and removal of ovaries you need to be careful about bone loss because the hormones secreted by the ovaries (and possibly aided by the uterus) are instrumental in preventing such loss. For reasons that remain unclear, progesterone, testosterone, and especially estrogen have a protective effect on the bones. Estrogen also keeps bones from losing calcium. Hormone replacement therapy can stave off further bone deterioration, but it cannot restore any previous loss.

Usually there are no early signs of osteoporosis. A bone breakage during a seemingly light fall may in fact be the first clue. Because it's a progressive disease, detection at an early stage can prevent further damage. There are tests you can talk to your doctor about, but gradual bone loss is difficult to pick up, even with X rays. A number of osteoporosis centers where bone-density X rays are taken have sprung up in recent years. There has, however, been some controversy about these because their diagnoses are not always 100 percent accurate.

There are ways you can insure maximum bone health. One is by paying attention to diet. Calcium, as the media and advertisements have undoubtedly informed you, is key. A minimum of 1,500 milligrams daily is recommended. If you don't get this through your present diet, consider taking supplements. Your diet should also include sufficient quantities of vitamin D, which promotes the absorption of calcium. Moderation—in all areas of diet—is important. Too much vitamin D actually aggravates bone thinning. An excess of salt, coffee, or even dietary fiber can hinder the bone-building process as well. There are also certain medications with negative effects on the bones. You can ask your physician if this could be a factor for you.

Exercise maximizes bone strength and density, and stimulates blood flow to the bones. The best exercises for bone strength are weight-bearing activities, such as jogging and walking. If bone attenuation has already begun, you can devise a program with your doctor's advice, since you don't want to overstrain your bones with high-impact exercise. It's also important not to smoke. Cigarettes seem to hinder estrogen metabolism and the blood cells are less effective in absorbing oxygen. Too much alcohol, too, gets in the way of calcium absorption.

Other preventative measures include hormone replacement therapy, as we've mentioned. Treatment of women for whom HRT is not an option and who already have some bone loss might include fluoride or the hormone calcitonin. This, however, requires careful monitoring by a physician.

Osteoporosis is a serious problem for women. The bone breaks that can result may leave someone bedridden or even incapacitated for the rest of her life. As with many disorders that catch public interest at a particular time, misconceptions about the problem abound. Get the best information you can on it and be wary of highly touted treatments. Not every supplement is effective, so you should consult a medical professional before staking the health of your bones on it.

CHAPTER 11

Sex After Hysterectomy

Possibly the most common question asked about hysterectomy is, Will it affect my sex life? For those who have turned to this chapter hoping for a definitive answer, there is unfortunately no clear-cut response. Some women, for reasons discussed later in this chapter, do find their libido lagging a bit compared to how they felt before the operation. Others, however, feel their enjoyment of sex has undoubtedly improved. This is especially true of women whose fibroids, endometriosis, or other conditions have made sex uncomfortable or painful for them in the past.

Sexuality is a complex part of a woman, an individual's sexual response being a blend of physiological and emotional factors. A disruption in either the physical or emotional can throw things out of kilter for a spell. Hysterectomy, as we've seen, can affect both—and so it stands to reason that someone emerging from the operation may not feel her sexual self for a while. Depending on personal circumstances, some of these changes may be permanent; others may merely require some adjusting to. In any case, a hysterectomy does not herald the end of one's sex life.

It's understandable that a woman undergoing a hysterectomy would be fearful and ambivalent about sex after the operation. All the more reason you should discuss this ahead of time with your doctor, your partner, or a counselor. If you feel awkward broaching the subject with your physician, perhaps there's another health-care professional you can speak with. Many women are uncomfortable discussing their feelings about sex. To some it may seem trivial in the context of major hospital surgery; to others it may simply seem crass. But our sexuality is an integral part of who we are and how we feel, and any change in it is something we have to live with.

It's important to understand what is likely to happen before it actually occurs, because expectations alone can influence how you adjust. If you expect to jump back into an active sex life, you might be dismayed to find you just don't feel up to it. If you—and your partner—have accepted the fact that you might feel run-down for a while, neither will be likely to feel too unnerved about it. There are other effects you might be able to anticipate. If your hysterectomy propels you into an early menopause, for instance, you might have to reconcile yourself to certain repercussions of the hormonal shift.

The question of sex after hysterectomy is a somewhat controversial one, chiefly because medical professionals have for so long denied that the operation has any adverse effect on sex. The standard textbook view— which, you should realize, many physicians still adhere to—was that there was no reason for a woman's sexual experience to be any different after a hysterectomy. The correlary to this, sometimes stated, sometimes not, was that any perceived changes were the result of a psychological maladjustment on the woman's part. In this atmosphere, women who did experience a change were made to feel they were crazy in addition to having to cope with their new sense of sexuality.

In part, this party line was an effort to reassure women. But there was also a long-held misunderstanding about female sexuality. From the standpoint of the medical community, the woman's experience of sex was not the issue. The point was, could she *function* sexually? Or, put another way, could she participate in the act of intercourse? Since she could, it was deemed a nonissue. That sex and hysterectomy were not always considered from the woman's viewpoint is also reflected by the fact that a century ago removing the uterus was seen as a cure for a woman's excessive (and at that time, *excessive* meant merely that it existed) sex drive.

We should also consider that in recent decades sexual research has focused on the clitoris as the female center for sexual pleasure. (This is opposed to Freud's day, when a clitoral orgasm was derided as "immature"; a vaginal orgasm was deemed a sign of female sexual adjustment—never mind that most women experience orgasm clitorally.) It is only now that the uterus and cervix are recognized as being instrumental to many women's pleasurable experience during sex, and these women do lose an important site of sensation after a hysterectomy.

Fortunately, views about women and sex have changed. Sex today is regarded not simply as a means of generating babies but as something that greatly contributes to a person's self-esteem, health, and vitality. Our expectations concerning sex also differ today. This is no longer an activity suited only to those in their reproductive years; rather, we anticipate being sexually active throughout our lives. Since a woman who has a hysterectomy can plan to have many sexually active years ahead of her, how her operation will affect her sex life is certainly a pertinent question.

In the last several years there have been a number of studies of sex after hysterectomy. A few have shown that between one third and one half of post-hysterectomy patients do experience some decrease in interest and satisfaction in their sex lives. Such studies cannot always be taken on face value, however, because many studies have asked their subjects to remember how it was before surgery and then compare, which does not always generate an accurate response. Perhaps it is safest to state that many women do perceive a letdown, but it is overall a highly individual issue.

THE SHORT-TERM CHANGES

First, we'll look at what you can expect in the short run. For the very short run what you can expect is no sex. Your doctor may advise you specifically, but the general recommendation is that anyone who has a hysterectomy should wait at least four to six weeks before having intercourse. This is to minimize the risk of infection in the early recuperative period.

As you reach the close of this block of time, rather than feeling that you're ready to jump at the opportunity, you may feel apprehensive at the very prospect of sex. Many women are concerned that they'll hurt something or perhaps tear their stitches. It's highly unlikely that this will happen, but you can check with your doctor if you have any doubts that you've healed.

Other women may feel afraid that their bodies have changed, that they're "different." Accept that you have these feelings and give yourself time to work them out. Don't feel that you're in any way being "tested" by those first renewed attempts at sex. Reflect back on the first times you ever had sex and remember that it probably took a while for it to feel right. Also, you may recall that fear about sex left your muscles tense and made sex itself more difficult.

Expect that it can take a couple of months before intercourse feels wholly comfortable. Your vaginal tissue becomes thinner and more fragile when it's not used, and it needs to rebuild gradually. You can try different positions to see which causes the least discomfort. At the same time, you should realize that sex doesn't necessarily begin and end with intercourse. Sharing other physical affection and closeness with your partner is at least as important in renewing your sexual bond.

Another reason you may not feel up to sexual par in the initial months after surgery is pure and simple exhaustion. Just as you probably don't feel terribly frisky when you're recovering from a bad flu, the fatigue that can ensue following a hysterectomy may curtail the energy you'd have for sex. Again, instead of concluding that this proves the hysterectomy has changed you and that your sex life will never be the same, just accept that this is a predictable outcome and that as the rest of you gets back in gear your sexuality will too.

Now we'll explore some factors that could produce changes in sexuality after hysterectomy—as well as some suggestions on how to cope with them.

PSYCHOLOGICAL FACTORS

When it comes to sexuality, the body is not a machine whose response can be scheduled or programmed at will. For instance, sexuality can often act as a barometer in a relationship; the first hint of discord or uncertainty in a romance generally reveals itself in bed. In the same way, someone's own emotional state greatly affects that person's sex life. The enjoyment of sex is in many ways a celebration of good feeling, and if one is feeling there's not much to celebrate, the pleasure taken in sex may wane.

For this reason, if a woman is experiencing some depression or confusion about herself after a hysterectomy, her sex life is going to reflect it. Sometimes a woman finds her sense of femininity altered by losing her uterus. She may feel that the absence of the uterus makes her less of a woman. As a result, she may feel sexually unattractive and may on a deeper level feel that it's not appropriate for her to be sexual anymore. Often, merely recognizing that this concern is hindering your sexual receptiveness can help you confront the issue and get beyond it. But if such beliefs seem to be deep-rooted, it may be advisable to seek counseling.

With other women the prime concern is not the uterus itself but its connection to childbearing. Many women's sexual identity is closely tied to their ability to have children. Younger women who suddenly find the option of having a baby taken away from them quite commonly experience this reaction. Even if they've already had the number of children they wanted or even if they didn't actually want to be mothers, the abrupt loss of the *possibility* of subsequent births can be quite devastating.

With both of these scenarios, it's important to note that such feelings may crop up unannounced; you may not realize that the potential to have a baby has a profound meaning to you until that potential is withdrawn. It's not always possible to predict how a given woman will respond, so it helps to be prepared for the type of reactions that might occur. It is also a good idea to have an understanding of what your uterus and childbearing capacity mean to you before you have the hysterectomy. Had she done this, Sandra might have been better able to handle the sexual shake-up that took place after her operation.

Sandra had just turned thirty-two when she learned she had cancer in situ of the cervix. She already had two children, which was all she and her husband wanted, and had been considering having her tubes tied. So although she realized there were alternative treatments to a hysterectomy—her doctor suggested having a cone biopsy and then following her for subsequent signs of disease—she decided to go ahead with the hysterectomy. She thought this would be easier, taking care of two problems with one sweep, and didn't like the notion of having "abnormal cells" in her body, despite her doctor's reassurances.

About two or three months after the hysterectomy, Sandra found herself growing wistful. She watched her children getting bigger and was sorry that they'd never be infants again. These feelings surprised her; she had a boy and a girl and hadn't had any desire for any more. She felt depressed and completely uninterested in sex. In all of her married life, she had either been trying to get pregnant or actively trying to avoid it. Either way, her fertility had never been far from her mind. Without it, sex just didn't seem right.

Sandra's husband was very supportive about this and suggested she see a therapist. With counseling, she was able to work through her loss, and fully appreciate the family life she did have.

Sometimes a woman is primarily afraid of her partner's reaction, wondering whether *he'll* continue to find her attractive after the operation. This may even lead her to shut down physically to insure that he won't approach her sexually and possibly be disappointed with her. Again, it would help to have a sense of what the operation and any potential changes might mean to him.

Talking about the issue, no matter how reluctant to do so you might be, is essential. If he seems shy of initiating sex, it could be that he's afraid of hurting you or thinks you're physically not ready for inter-course. In this case, you need only allay his fears. It's also possible that you're assuming it's a reaction against your femininity when in fact *he's* having doubts about his own masculinity. Just as women are affected by the loss of fertility, men can feel that their manhood is threatened by the inability to have a child—regardless of the source. Communication can help both of you cope with the confusing emotions the hysterectomy may trigger.

HORMONAL FACTORS

Hormones are the chemicals our body makes to trigger many vital responses. In many ways they drive human sexuality: the hormones produced in the ovaries give a woman her femininity; those generated in the testes give a man his masculine qualities. Sexual arousal and activity also depend on the secretion of these substances.

Our endocrine system, of which hormones are a part, is extremely complex, and hormones circulate through our bodies according to a delicately balanced plan. The ovaries—and as we've recently discovered, the uterus—are tied in with this system, so it stands to reason that anything affecting either or both of them would in turn have an impact on sexuality.

The ovaries produce the estrogens that surge and wane to produce the menstrual cycle. Estrogen affects other bodily functions, and can influence skin smoothness and elasticity, sexual capacity, and a sense of well-being. Progesterone, also made in the ovaries, similarly rises and falls in a cyclical pattern. Androgens, including testosterone, are ovarian hormones as well (although some quantities are produced in the adrenal glands). While they occur in both sexes, androgens are often called "male hormones" because they're found in higher levels in men and produce many male secondary characteristics including beard growth, muscular development, and a deepened voice. In women, androgens play a large role in sex drive.

Until recently, the uterus was not thought to be significant in terms of hormones, but it has been established that uterine substances are instrumental in keeping the ovaries manufacturing and secreting them. In the same way, the hormonal function of the ovaries was considered inconsequential in postmenopausal women. It now seems clear that both the ovaries and the uterus are involved in processes that can affect a woman's sexuality—throughout her life.

When a woman loses her ovaries, this causes hormonal shifts that can alter her sex life considerably. This is particularly true of women in their childbearing years; they are suddenly catapulted into menopause and thus experience, in a particularly dramatic way, all the sexual changes that come with menopause. The level of androgens plummets. The vaginal walls may become drier and thinner, often making sex uncomfortable. In addition, the lowered level of estrogen in the vagina alters the vagina's acidity. As a result, such women may be prone to yeast infections. While yeast infections don't make sex impossible, they can certainly make it less pleasant.

Pheromones, chemical secretions that are thought to be perceived as "odors" involved in sexual attraction, are also likely to be altered. While much remains to be learned about these substances, it's possible that any changes could alter a woman's sexual appeal to men as well as her sexual responses to them.

With the menstrual cycle no longer in operation, the rise and fall of sexual interest that goes along with it will disappear. For some women this may have a stabilizing quality and they'll appreciate the fact that they can have sex at any point in the cycle, but others may miss their regular rhythms of desire.

Women who have chosen to have their ovaries left in may experience some of these changes as well. First of all, the blood supply to the ovaries may have been altered by the hysterectomy, which can affect their ability to produce and secrete hormones. And second, the removal of the uterus may inhibit the ovaries' functioning.

Hormone therapies can address many of these changes, but they can never replace the natural hormones 100 percent. Androgen replacement therapy has been used to help revive sexual appetite, but this can carry with it some unpleasant side effects, specifically masculinizing ones like the growth of facial hair, increased oiliness in the skin (which can cause acne), and a lowered voice. One androgen delivery system under investigation that is hoped to cause fewer side effects is a slow-release pellet inserted under the skin at the hip.

Many of the hormonal upsets do subside with time, as the body merely adjusts to its new rhythms. Remember also that sexuality evolves naturally as one ages. If, however, you're finding the post-hysterectomy changes to be quite drastic, you should definitely discuss the possible treatments with your physician.

The body's hormones also interact with sexuality the other way around. Your sexual behavior can influence your pattern of hormone production. Women who have found that their own menstrual patterns have fallen in sync with their close friends' have witnessed something similar to this phenomenon: that our hormonal cycles can be swayed by external factors.

In her book *Hysterectomy: Before & After*, Winnifred B. Cutler, Ph.D., describes research that found that women who engaged in regular sex with a male partner had higher levels of estrogen (though within the normal range) and greater menstrual regularity than women who didn't. These particular effects are often associated with greater fertility. Women who were celibate or whose sex lives were off and on had estrogen levels and patterns of basal body temperature that tended to reflect lowered fertility. The point is that an active sex life can keep hormone production active as well. The closer to par your hormone levels are, the more sexually responsive you're able to be, both before the operation and after.

OTHER PHYSICAL EFFECTS

A hysterectomy can prompt other physical changes that may affect a woman's experience of sex. Women who have had their ovaries removed will find their vaginal lubrication diminished. This can generally be remedied by using a lubricant, but some women may be a bit thrown off by the sudden change. After all, vaginal lubrication is part of a woman's sexual response and it signals arousal, much like a man's erection. Estrogen replacement therapy may restore some moistness (especially if it's administered locally—see Chapter 12 on ERT), but basically it's something that has to be gotten used to.

There are possible local effects from surgery. Certain nerves that contribute to sexual sensation or blood vessels that affect hormone production could be intruded on by the surgical process. This seems to pose less of a problem with a supracervical hysterectomy; greater problems are seen with vaginal hysterectomies.

In some instances the vagina will be shortened by a hysterectomy. This could occur after a vaginal hysterectomy done for uterine prolapse (in which case the vagina may be narrowed as well) or following a hysterectomy to treat cancer, during which part of the top of the vagina may have been removed to prevent the spread of malignancy. Radiation therapy for cancer can also affect the elasticity and wetness of the vagina.

These changes in the vagina can make intercourse uncomfortable and in extreme cases could render penile penetration impossible. Scar tissue in the pelvis or at the top of the vagina can also interfere with sex and make it painful. Other complications, such as a wound or bladder infection, could likewise cause pain during sexual intercourse. Sometimes such effects are temporary or require further treatment; sometimes they persist.

A hysterectomy may disrupt the sex lives of some women more than others—depending on where and how they experience pleasure. For the vast majority of women, orgasm is felt in the lower vagina and the clitoral region, and a hysterectomy does not change this. Some women, however, derive pleasure from deep sensations within the uterus. The cervix itself is rich with nerve endings and some women may be brought to orgasm by the penis or fingers pressing against the cervix and uterus. Such feelings will be lost after hysterectomy. Some women report having an "empty feeling" during sex following the operation.

If you try to think about it or try to focus on your physical sensations when you have sex, you can probably determine whether your pleasure would be affected. If your sexual pleasure does depend on feelings centered in the cervix or uterus and you fear your sex life will suffer as a result, you can discuss the possibility of a supracervical hysterectomy with your doctor. On the other hand, if you realize that your orgasms are generally clitoral-based, you can be reassured that you are not likely to lose much sensation there.

The uterus, as we have seen, is not a sexually inert organ. It is involved in all phases of the sexual process: desire, arousal, and orgasm. The ovarian hormones it helps to stimulate have an effect on desire. During arousal, the uterus helps to promote lubrication and it swells up and becomes engorged with blood—all of which moves the body toward a peak of excitement. And, during orgasm, the uterus contracts in a rhythm comparable to the man's climax.

Depending on the woman, the post-hysterectomy sexual changes may be significant or barely noticeable at all. And for lots of women, a hysterectomy gives their sexual lives a lift. This is especially true of those who suffered from conditions that had slowed them down sexually. Women with severe endometriosis, for instance, will feel greatly liberated by the fact that they can now have sex without pain. The same holds true for a number of other problems.

Marcia, forty-five, was an observant Orthodox Jew, which meant she was not allowed to have sexual intercourse during the time she was bleeding and the week after. For many women, this religious restriction required forgoing sex for just those two weeks. But because Marcia consistently had heavy bleeding for at least two weeks out of the month, she virtually couldn't have sex at all.

After her hysterectomy, Marcia said she'd never felt better. In her words, she "felt like a human being again." The blood loss had made her anemic, and there were times she couldn't go out of the house. With the bleeding no longer a problem, she and her husband were able to have the healthy sexual relationship they had before the bleeding had started.

Even without such religious restrictions, many women with excessive bleeding are quite uncomfortable with intercourse. They find themselves thinking more about the bleeding and staining of the sheets than of the activity in bed. A woman with pelvic pain or endometriosis often feels the same way. She becomes afraid of the pain and less interested in sex; her partner then fears causing her more pain and stops making any overtures. A hysterectomy that relieves the pain or bleeding can break the cycle that had pretty much brought their sexual relationship to a halt.

Other women have felt burdened by the constant bother of contraception and may revel in their new sexual freedom. For women whose hysterectomies were medically essential, the sexual loss is often minimal. If someone's life has been threatened by cancer and now she is all right, the potential effects on sex seem but a small price to pay. For women who undergo hysterectomy by choice, the loss may loom larger.

Some of these changes in sex after hysterectomy may happen to you, and in many instances you will learn to live with them. But there are things you can do. Regular sex helps stir up hormone production, as mentioned earlier in the chapter. But remember that this also includes sexual play that stops short of intercourse. You and your partner can be more creative with your sex lives and not always focus on intercourse as the inevitable finale. You can experiment more with oral sex, varying positions, and taking the whole thing *slower* to give yourself a chance to lubricate naturally. For women without regular partners, masturbation helps. It increases blood flow to the region and helps keep your muscles in shape. Pelvic exercises are also beneficial.

An active sex life unquestionably enhances your state of mind and your health. A hysterectomy does not need to slow down your sex life, but you may have to give it a bit more work than you're used to. Not all women are completely comfortable with all of these issues, but taking responsibility for your own sexuality is a very positive step for anyone—despite many of the hang-ups we were raised with or have accumulated on our own.

CHAPTER 12

The Question of Hormone Therapy

There was a time, about twenty years ago, when the medical community thought it had discovered the fountain of youth. Wrinkle-free skin, renewed sexual vigor, health and vitality—this is what postmenopausal women were told they could expect with estrogen therapy. Then, in the mid-1970s, a disturbing trend was noticed: the occurence of certain cancers was creeping up, and this seemed to be associated with the widespread use of estrogen. As suddenly as estrogen's popularity had soared, its use began to plummet. Alarmed by the cancer statistics, many women came to regard estrogen replacement therapy as something to avoid.

When it comes to putting any substance in your body, medically or otherwise, a degree of cynicism can be a good thing. In the case of estrogen therapy, a good deal has been learned in the past few decades about both the risks it presents and how those risks can be minimized. It's therefore best to base your decision on what the most up-to-date therapies can offer you and how they fit in with your own health needs.

The reason for the rise in cancer rates is that certain cancers, primarily endometrial cancer (see Chapter 6 on endometrial hyperplasia), can be promoted by high levels of estrogen. Also, in earlier years the estrogen was prescribed in high doses, on the assumption that the more a woman took, the younger she would feel. Recently, however, the dosage has been cut way back. Today most treatments will also include progestins, which serve to balance out the estrogen levels and neutralize the negative effects excess estrogen can have on the uterine lining. As a result, the cancer rates have flattened out and the treatment has gotten safer in general. The more that is learned about hormones, the closer the therapies get to the balance that would occur naturally.

Another reason hormone replacement therapy (HRT) has been controversial is that there are two opposing views within the medical community. One takes the stand that a woman's "normal" hormonal state is that of her childbearing years. Menopause thus needs to be regarded as a diseased state and treated with the appropriate hormones. The other faction maintains that since estrogens naturally diminish with the onset of menopause, this hormonal condition should be accepted as normal. Treatment, then, would be recommended when there are indications other than mere aging.

Women today can look forward to many healthy years after menopause. When life expectancy was much shorter, the long-term consequences of postmenopausal estrogen loss, such as osteoporosis, vaginal dryness, and possibly cardiovascular disease, would not have been an issue. But now the question of hormone therapy is a highly relevant issue for every woman. Women do have reason for concern—and reason to be informed—because many doctors prescribe HRT more or less automatically. Also, there are still unanswered questions regarding its long-term effects, especially after extended periods of usage. And many women take hormonal therapies for a long time, notably those who have had hysterectomies at a relatively young age.

Hormone replacement therapy can be a boost to a woman's health. To determine the best course, each woman should, in conjunction with her doctor, carefully evaluate risks, benefits, and alternatives. HRT is a form of therapy that can be highly individualized, so you can arrive at an appropriate treatment with minimal short- and long-term effects.

At the age of fifty-three, when she was pretty well through her natural menopause, Carole had a hysterectomy with bilateral oophorectomy. The reason for the operation had been fibroids, so she was considered eligible for HRT. Her older sister, however, had recently been diagnosed with breast cancer, and Carole emphatically informed her doctor that she did not want any hormone treatment.

She went without treatment for about six months but wasn't feeling well at all. She had vaginal dryness that paralyzed her sex life, and she felt dragged down by a depression she couldn't seem to shake. At that point her doctor suggested an estrogen skin patch. The patch left an irritation on her skin, but at this point she decided she was ready to explore other forms of HRT. After trying low-dose estrogen pills for a while, she finally felt back to normal. Carole was still less than completely comfortable with the idea of taking estrogen, but she does monthly breast self-exams and has regular mammograms to insure that no lumps develop.

THE BENEFITS

The most immediately apparent benefits of hormonal replacement therapy are in managing menopausal symptoms. Night sweats, hot flashes, vaginal dryness, emotional swings—all should be minimized by the treatment. Lots of women take HRT as a stopgap to carry them through a period of severe menopausal symptoms. Although not the magical formula for perpetual youth it was once touted to be, HRT does fill out wrinkles and make skin look younger. This is partly because it increases water retention, but also that it stimulates the growth of skin cells.

HRT is most important in preventing osteoporosis, which begins to wear away women's bones in the years succeeding menopause. The greatest benefit is usually derived by women who take HRT for several years past the age of natural menopause, which on average today is age fifty-one. Premenopausal women who have hysterectomies, however, may begin the treatment at a much earlier age. HRT can't restore lost bone, but if it is applied in the years immediately following menopause, there can be some improvement. HRT also minimizes further bone deterioration. Women who already show signs of osteoporosis are generally advised to be on some HRT program, unless there are strong medical reasons prohibiting it, in which case alternative treatments can be considered.

Hormonal treatments can also be a boon to cardiovascular health. This makes sense, because before menopause, when estrogen production remains consistently high, women suffer from heart disease at a much lower rate than men, who lack the protection of estrogen. The precise reason for this, however, remains unclear. It does seem that supplementary estrogen lowers the heart attack risk among young women who have had their ovaries removed, although the correlation among older women is less pronounced. There is evidence that estrogen plays a role in the way cholesterol is metabolized and somehow deters the rise of LDL, which is the "bad" form of cholesterol that contributes to the buildup of fats in the arteries. Some research indicates, however, that with progestins, which have a moderating effect on estrogen, the cardiovascular benefits are diminished.

Note that with cardiovascular health, as well as with bone strength, the HRT is merely part of the regimen; only by combining it with your nutrition and fitness efforts are you doing your best to reach optimal health.

Another possible benefit of HRT is that it can help prevent rheumatoid arthritis. The estrogen can reduce the inflammation that damages the joint. Indeed, it is common for women to get vague joint pain around the time of menopause that seems to be relieved by HRT.

The treatment may also lower the instance of urinary tract infections, which tend to occur with increasing frequency and persistency after menopause, when tissue in the bladder and the urethra loses its elasticity. There are indications that HRT also enhances muscle tone and has a positive effect on the immune system.

A woman who has lost her ovaries during a hysterectomy may want to consider taking androgens, which are the hormones that have the greatest effect on libido. In women, these male hormones are produced both in the ovaries and in the adrenal glands. It had been thought that estrogen replacement alone would restore libido after ovary removal, but the only effect it appears to have on lagging sexuality is to clear up the menopausal symptoms that adversely affect sex, including vaginal dryness and the thinning of the vaginal walls, both of which can make sex uncomfortable.

It's important to note that the benefits of HRT last only as long as the medications are taken. So someone who is doing well on them will probably take them for the rest of her life.

THE RISKS

The two major risks of hormonal therapy are endometrial cancer and breast cancer. Medical authorities are in conflict as to whether or not the actual incidence of disease is increased, but theoretically if a woman was predisposed to develop breast cancer, for example, the development of abnormal cells may be accelerated and may occur at an earlier age.

Someone who has had a hysterectomy will, of course, not be at risk of uterine cancer. The rise in the rate of breast cancer has not been completely confirmed, but is worrisome on a theoretical basis. One recent study however, suggested that women on HRT who have lost their ovaries are at an elevated risk if they are between fifty and fifty-four years of age and have a close relative who has been diagnosed with breast cancer. In light of these concerns, any woman on hormonal therapy is generally advised to have a yearly mammogram.

The progestin that is commonly added to estrogen in treatment is generally intended to protect the uterus from precancerous changes. If a woman has had a hysterectomy, however, the need for progestin is less clear. In one recent study, it was shown to increase the risk of breast cancer. It could also cause unpleasant side effects, such as headaches or depression, as well as compromise the healthful effects estrogen has on the accumulation of lipids in the arteries. Also, progestins have not been studied to the extent that estrogens have, so other negative effects associated with progestin may yet emerge.

Nor is androgen therapy without its potential problems. The main trouble here is its possible masculinizing effects, including excessive hair growth, acne, a lower-pitched voice, and an enlargement of the clitoris. If any of these should arise, alert your physician and you will probably be put on a reduced dosage or taken off androgens altogether. As with progestins, the long-term effects on women who take androgen have not been determined.

Because of the side effects prompted by hormonal therapies, all women taking hormones should be sure to schedule regular medical checkups. The estrogen itself has been known to trigger a host of problems, such as nausea, vomiting, bloating, weight gain, breast swelling and tenderness, headaches, and bleeding. These are less likely to occur today because of the lowered doses in use, and many symptoms tend to recede on their own. Weight gain and bloating, for instance, are primarily a result of excess water retention, which should correct itself within a few months.

HRT comes in so many forms and can be administered in such a variety of dosages that side effects can usually be diminished by simply adjusting the prescription. If you find yourself beset by any of these HRT-related problems, don't feel that you should simply stick it out. Let your doctor know, so you can experiment with the dosage or form to determine the best program for you. It often takes a few tries to get it just right. If you're bothered by breast soreness or bloating, the estrogen level may be too high, for example. It's often a good idea to make notes on the symptomatic

changes you experience and report these to your doctor
to facilitate the inevitable trial-and-error period.

There are many women for whom HRT is not even
an option. Someone who has had cancer of the endometrium or breast may not be a candidate for hormones.
Nor might someone who has a history of abnormal
clotting, as the possibility of estrogens having an effect
on clotting has been raised. Since clotting can occur
with pelvic surgery, anyone who has been on HRT
before the hysterectomy should check with her physician about suspending treatment for the period immediately preceding the operation. In addition, medications
for other problems may impact the hormonal balance,
so your doctor should be aware of anything else you're
taking.

Often, women who have had an estrogen-related
disorder, such as endometrial hyperplasia or cancer, are
discouraged from taking estrogens, but instead are put
on progestins. However, unopposed progestins will diminish the benefits that any remaining estrogen would
bring, thus leaving the body quite estrogen-deprived.
In the case of endometriosis, estrogen may not be prescribed after a hysterectomy for fear that the disease
may recur in whatever endometrial implants have been
left behind. Usually, delaying the start of estrogen therapy until six months or a year after surgery for endometriosis will reduce the chance of recurrence of disease.
Another point to keep in mind is that women, especially
those before the age of menopause, who retain their
ovaries may be producing sufficient estrogen on their
own and may not need additional therapy.

Hormone replacement therapies are dispensed in a number of forms. Estrogens can be natural or synthetic. Premarin, a commonly prescribed estrogen in pill form, is made from natural horse estrogens. Estradiol, on the other hand, is a manufactured synthetic. With progestins, only synthetics may be taken as a pill; natural progesterone would have to be taken as a vaginal suppository or injection. Natural progesterone is not widely available, nor do all women respond well to it. Androgen therapy is currently not very prevalent, but is occasionally used when problems with sex drive occur.

Estrogens can be taken in the form of pills, injections, creams, skin patches, or inserts placed under the skin. For women with liver disease, other forms of estrogen may be preferable to pills, which are metabolized in the liver. Anyone who has difficulty swallowing pills may similarly prefer other treatments. The patch, through which the medication is absorbed, is generally placed on the abdomen or buttocks and should be replaced twice a week. It also tends to be more expensive than many of the alternative forms.

Estrogen cream, which is inserted vaginally at a lower dosage than other forms, is often chosen by women who aren't particularly comfortable with the notion of taking hormones. Its effects are chiefly local: alleviating the problems of vaginal dryness and thinning vaginal walls. Some is absorbed into the bloodstream, but the extent is less predictable. As a result, the effectiveness of estrogen cream for treating osteoporosis or offering other benefits is questionable. Women who for medical reasons are not candidates for hormonal therapy will not be able to take estrogen this way either. The cream should not be used before intercourse, because it can rub off on the man's penis and he will absorb the hormones.

Pills have the advantage of being quick and simple to take. Also, progestins are nearly always administered in pill form, which might make it more convenient to take estrogen as pills too. Some women do, however, become nauseous as a result of the estrogen pills.

Other forms of estrogen include pills that are not swallowed but are placed under the tongue, injections, and a new type, pellets that are surgically inserted under the skin. None, however, are as prevalent as the pills, patch, or cream.

1

1 EP	2 EP	3 EP	4 EP	5 EP	6 EP	7 EP
8 EP	9 EP	10 EP	11 EP	12 EP	13 E	14 E
15 E	16 E	17 E	18 E	19 E	20 E	21 E
22 E	23 E	24 E	25 E	26 E	27 E	28 E

Continual Estrogen
Progesterone days 1–12
Period day 13

2

1 E	2 E	3 E	4 E	5 E	6 E	7 E
8 E	9 E	10 E	11 E	12 E	13 E	14 E
15 EP	16 EP	17 EP	18 EP	19 EP	20 EP	21 EP
22	23	24	25	26	27	28

Estrogen 3 weeks on, 1 week off
Progesterone last week of estrogen
Period day 22, 23, or 24

3						
1 P	2 EP	3 P	4 P	5 EP	6 P	7 P
8 P	9 EP	10 P	11 P	12 EP	13	14
15	16 E	17	18	19 E	20	21
22	23 E	24	25	26 E	27	28

Estrogen patch 2 times a week
Progesterone days 1–12
Period day 13 or 14

4						
1 E	2 E	3 E	4 E	5 E	6 E	7 E
8 E	9 E	10 E	11 E	12 E	13 E	14 E
15 E	16 EP	17 EP	18 EP	19 EP	20 EP	21 EP
22 EP	23 EP	24 EP	25 EP	26	27	28

Estrogen days 1–25
Progesterone days 16–25
Period day 26 or 27
Here, even though there are no hormones at the end of the
month, the hormones still stay in the body (when in pill form).

5

1	2 E	3	4	5 E	6	7
8	9 E	10	11	12 E	13	14
15	16 EP	17 P	18 P	19 EP	20 P	21 P
22 P	23 EP	24 P	25 P	26	27	28

Estrogen patch 2 times a week, days 1–25
Progesterone days 16–25
Period day 26 or 27
Hot flashes may occur when off hormones.

6

1 EP	2 EP	3 EP	4 EP	5 EP	6 EP	7 EP
8 EP	9 EP	10 EP	11 EP	12 EP	13 EP	14 EP
15 EP	16 EP	17 EP	18 EP	19 EP	20 EP	21 EP
22 EP	23 EP	24 EP	25 EP	26 EP	27 EP	28 EP

For women who don't want any bleeding
Estrogen every day
Progesterone small dose every day
(Irregular bleeding first three months, then no bleeding
thereafter.)

CHAPTER 13

Taking Charge of Making the Decision

With the rare exception, there is no *immediate* need to decide about a hysterectomy. That means there is ample time for a second opinion, to explore other treatment options, and get all the information you need to obtain from your doctor or any other sources. You should not feel *pressured* to put your name on the schedule for surgery.

The decision to have a hysterectomy should always be made in cooperation with your doctor, not in spite of your doctor and certainly not in complete deference to your doctor. Your relationship with your doctor, then, needs to be a cooperative one, not an adversarial one and not a passive one.

Having a doctor should not mean turning over total responsibility for your health to another person. Sometimes we want to simply put ourselves in the doctor's hands and let him or her take care of everything. But playing an active part in decisions about your health is ultimately empowering to you as a patient. Understanding what lies ahead of you will reduce the stress associated with anticipating surgery. A number of recent studies have shown that when people feel powerless and at the mercy of others, their ability to recuperate from illness or surgery is compromised. By being informed and confident of your decision, you're putting yourself in a position of strength.

A hysterectomy is something you live with for the rest of your life, so you need a doctor who is willing and able to discuss personal and emotional factors as well as strictly medical ones. Many women hesitate to discuss such issues as how the operation may affect their sex lives, how their partners will react, and how to deal with the emotional swings that may accompany hormonal changes. To some, it seems inappropriate to bring up intimate matters in a clinical setting— and with someone who is a virtual stranger and possibly male. But it's not only appropriate to do so, it's necessary in order to maintain your health and well-being. Better to clarify the emotional realities before the operation than to allow them to sneak up on you later.

The initial step in working with your doctor is, of course, finding a doctor you feel you can work with comfortably. It's important to keep in mind that you're not stuck with a given doctor or legally bound to a medical provider who has helped you in the past. If you already have a gynecologist you're happy with, that's great. But if you're not pleased with your doctor's treatment or approach, you should feel free to look elsewhere.

In seeking out a new doctor, either upon moving into a community or replacing one that didn't suit you, you need above all to consider medical competence and expertise. Make sure that the doctor has been certified by the American Board of Obstetrics and Gynecology. This alone is no guarantee of excellence, but it suggests some level of proficiency and training. It's also helpful to check with local sources, such as the county medical society, a family doctor, or friends. You can't simply take reputation on face value, however, for you don't always know just how that reputation was built. A doctor may be renowned as an ace in the operating room, for instance. But if he or she has earned that fame by being ready to don surgical gloves at the drop of a hat—or the first drop of blood—that doesn't necessarily bode well for your health.

Nor does the fact that a friend thinks the world of a certain doctor mean this is the doctor for you. Your chemistry with a professional may be different than someone else's. Some women may feel more at ease with a female gynecologist; others may prefer a male one. You may like a doctor with a more open style; someone else may choose one who's more businesslike.

You should go into your first or any meeting with a doctor with an open mind. Because, just as in any interpersonal relationship, you have to work at it—and it takes both people involved to make it work. If you find, for example, that you appreciate some aspects of your doctor's care but are wary of others, you can raise those issues and see if you can work things out so that you're comfortable. If you feel your doctor is technically competent but you find that he or she rushes and doesn't explain procedures fully, you could make it a point to ask specific questions and take it upon yourself to understand everything before he or she proceeds. If your doctor is not willing to work with you or actively discourages you from getting a second opinion, you'd probably be wise to consider a switch.

Keep in mind that any question that goes unasked, also goes unanswered. It's not always the doctor's fault that the patient doesn't know something. You can't expect your doctor to be a mind reader. No one can know what you need to hear until you tell him. So it's up to you to state your concerns and raise any issues you want addressed. Don't be reluctant to learn more about your condition because you're afraid to find out. We all cling to a superstitious belief that by not giving voice to a problem, it won't occur. When it comes to your health, ignorance is no protection.

Financial arrangements need to be discussed up front. Many women hesitate to bring up money questions, often because they fear it puts them in a bad light or because they're not comfortable about dealing with money issues in general. Few women would buy a car or even a pair of shoes without determining the price ahead of time, but how many consent to surgery without finding out how it may impact them financially?

In a preoperative visit you should ask the physician what the charges will be. Then check with your insurance company to see precisely what's covered. Many alternative treatments that involve less surgery are at least as expensive as hysterectomy because they may require special skills. Some newer procedures may not be covered at all. You can't assume that less time in the hospital will result in a lower medical bill.

It's important that you prepare yourself for the financial reality. Even the best insurance plans generally pay no more than 80 percent. If you work, check to see if your employer makes any provisions. If the cost is in the way, be up-front with your physician. Perhaps the fee can be cut or surgery can be arranged in a clinic. In some cases, an area physician may be conducting research at a medical center on hysterectomies or related operations. Your doctor would be the logical resource for finding the best possible alternative at a lower cost—far better than your going out on your own.

Whether the issue is financial or physical, for effective communication to take place you and your doctor need to be speaking the same language. Many doctors are used to talking primarily with other doctors, so a lot of jargon can get tossed around. If you don't grasp something he or she tells you, back up and keep inquiring until you're confident that you do understand. Don't ever feel embarrassed to ask the doctor to elaborate on a point because you think you *should* have caught it all the first time.

So many women seem to forget that their relationship with doctors is based on the fact that the doctor provides a service. Women who would automatically expect promptness, fairness, and respect from any other professional providing a service routinely shy away from "troubling" their physicians with complaints or concerns. But it's your doctor's job to deal with matters of your health. Your health and comfort should be important to your doctor, and it should be important enough to *you* to make certain you get the best care.

Rather than bothering your doctor, your questions probably please him or her. Most doctors prefer patients who are informed and who take an active interest in their own health. It's a lonely role to be asked to fix up a body whose owner shows no regard for it. Doctors constantly face patients who fail to take medication for the full cycle or are racked by a cough yet continue to smoke. So your doctor should be happy to help you understand what's happening to your body, since that suggests there may be fewer *mis*understandings and other problems down the line.

Soon after she learned she was going to have a hysterectomy, Sharon confessed to a friend that she was a nervous wreck about the whole thing. She had just started dating a man seriously and was worried about how he'd respond to it and whether it would affect their sex life. She wondered about how much time she'd be away from work and what kind of anesthesia she'd have.

"These are all questions you should be asking your doctor, not me," her friend said. At her friend's urging, Sharon revealed these concerns at her next appointment. The doctor spent a good half hour detailing aspects of the operation, and by the time Sharon left, she felt much more confident about the ordeal. She also felt

a new respect for her physician, who now seemed much more real a person. It occurred to her that she had always assumed her doctor, a quiet, gray-haired man, was cold and too busy, chiefly because she had never initiated any more personal interaction.

Yet "doctor phobia" persists, so it may help to get a sense of the source of it. For one thing, doctors are often viewed as a breed apart, as members of some elite and exclusive club. Most people are aware of the rigors of medical education and how competitive it is even to land a spot in medical school. It seems that they have special knowledge, as well as access to special machines and tools that give them power over the rest of us.

Then there are the circumstances under which your meetings with the doctor take place. You're stripped down to your underthings—or less—and he or she is fully dressed. That alone tends to make you feel vulnerable. You're in a stark, bright, not terribly comfortable room. You may have to wait, and there may or may not be nurses, lab technicians, or other health practitioners wandering in and out, scarcely acknowledging your existence. Your doctor will probably be busy, as doctors are generally busy, and you may feel the stress of this time pressure. Beyond all this is the fact that you're undoubtedly nervous about your health.

The point here is that it's important to get over doctor intimidation. A free exchange of information is especially important with an operation like hysterectomy because it is often a matter of judgment and because patients' experience of it and reaction to it vary so. In many cases, the doctor has little more to go on than the description of symptoms provided by the patient. A woman suffering from endometriosis, for example, may be in such agony that a hysterectomy is warranted. But if the same woman has a strong desire for children, it might be best for her to try to conceive (which, as seen in Chapter 5, can reduce the pain of endometriosis). The type of treatment she receives could depend on how she presents her situation to her physician.

So if you express a desperation to be freed of menstrual annoyance, a desire to be sterilized, or a terror of cancer, that's what your doctor will hear. Therefore, he or she will evaluate any physical findings in light of those concerns. Be open and explore other possible causes for your discomfort as you explore alternatives in treatment. Don't be so quick to assign a physical cause to a problem and then put all your hope in a physical resolution. It's often tempting to rely on surgery as the ultimate answer, especially if that problem has eluded all other attempted solutions. But, as we have seen, hysterectomy is rarely a simple cure for anything. It's important, then, not to jump into any decision and to be receptive to other factors. Sometimes, for instance, emotional stressors can affect the way we experience discomfort or the way our body reacts. Menstrual pain and menstrual bleeding both can be aggravated by stress, for example. Not all gynecologists are trained to track down emotional causes, and thus it is essential that you furnish as much information as you can.

The more knowledge you have about your own body and about hysterectomy, the better. Learn to identify changes in your body that may be relevant. Note when symptoms are most pronounced and when they ease up. It's often a good idea to take notes when you're speaking with your doctor, to enhance concentration and keep you from letting anything slip away. There's no need to feel silly or self-conscious about doing this. After all, the doctor has probably taken notes on your medical history. One possible way of handling the information-gathering phase is to have a friend or spouse sit in on your consultation. The extra support might make you feel more comfortable and freer to articulate your views.

It's also advisable to have a written list of questions that you're sure to want answered. This keeps the subject from getting too overwhelming and can help you organize your thoughts. Here, as a rough guide, is a list of possible questions:

- What is the reason for the recommended hysterectomy?
- Are there alternative treatments for this condition?
- If surgery is to be done, what exactly will be removed? Are there alternatives here?
- What type of incision will be used? Again, are there other options?
- Am I at a high risk for any particular complications?

- What are my chances of needing blood during the operation?
- Are there any treatments I will need in addition to the hysterectomy?
- What will be the cost?
- How long should I expect to be in the hospital? How long should I expect to be out of work?
- Are there ways I can prepare myself ahead of time?

A second opinion is not something you get only when you have reason to doubt the first doctor's advice. It's absolutely essential when you're dealing with a major operation. Some insurance companies, in fact, require that a recommendation for surgery be confirmed by a second source before any reimbursement. Many people are concerned that the original doctor might be offended by "second-guessing" his or her diagnosis, but it's certainly in everybody's best interest to have a clear course of action that all can accept.

During a routine pelvic exam, Margaret's doctor found a small solid mass on an ovary. Later, a sonogram confirmed that it was solid, and solid tumors are more likely to be malignant than others. She was only thirty-eight, an age when most ovarian tumors prove benign, but her doctor was concerned because it showed no signs of going away and urged her to have the ovary removed or the mass taken out. Margaret next went to see another doctor, a big shot at her area hospital whose opinions were widely respected. He said not to worry, that the tumor wasn't terribly large and might well subside on its own.

At this point Margaret felt confused. She had gone to this doctor specifically for his expert opinion, yet she wasn't sure it was right to follow it. She couldn't get out of her mind what the first doctor had said—that a solid mass meant a greater chance of malignancy—which had a compelling logic. The other doctor was soothing, yet somehow less convincing.

She went back to her initial doctor and had the operation. The tumor was indeed cancerous. Had she ignored the first doctor and gone instead with the second, the malignancy might have spread.

The point here is that you should do more than collect opinions from various doctors. You need to *listen* to what they say and to what their reasoning is. If the two opinions are split, and you're still not clear, you may even want to seek a third opinion. This you should choose very carefully. Consider consulting a specialist in the area: if the question involves cancer, see a cancer specialist (oncologist); if it's related to fertility, track down a fertility specialist. Or you may want to go to a medical center specialist. For such cases, don't simply visit the doctor your insurance company recommends.

With the rate of unnecessary hysterectomies thought to be so high, a second opinion is an important protective measure. Studies show that even the knowledge that every medical opinion will need confirmation lowers the rate of hysterectomies performed. According to Dr. Herbert Keyser in *Women Under the Knife*, a 30 percent nonconfirmation rate is typical when second opinions for hysterectomies are mandatory. More than half of these patients, he adds, proved able to avoid the surgery altogether.

For the second opinion, it's advisable to pick a doctor who has no affiliation with your current doctor. You may then choose to go outside the community if you live in a small city or town. A teaching hospital or university hospital can be a good bet. Dr. Keyser recommends following certain basic rules: first, that you inform the consulting doctor up front as to the purpose of your visit. Second, that it's preferable not to reveal the name of your original physician until the session is over. And last, that the consultant's role is *only* to recommend the best treatment and not to take part in any treatment. (In situations that require special medical expertise, however, this may not be the case.) This insures that the consultant has nothing to gain either way and can best maintain objectivity.

With hysterectomy, it's important that you not feel alone. Talk to friends and to other women you know who have been through it. Every woman's experience may be different, but everyone's experience is valid, and you're likely to learn a great deal from others. Also, simply knowing that you're not the only one that's been through this can be comforting and reassuring. Your husband or partner shouldn't be excluded from the process. He is going to be affected by the changes that affect you, so help his adjustment along by informing him about the facts of hysterectomy. He will be most able to support you when he understands what it is you're facing. And remember that emotional or couples' counseling is available if you need it.

Beyond your own private circle, there are support groups that can provide assistance and information. Ask the women's or health organizations in your community to point you in the right direction. Some organizations that either sponsor support groups or may be able to refer you to one include:

- Hysterectomy Educational Resources and Services (HERS) Foundation
- Endometriosis Association
- Resolve
- Planned Parenthood

For Further Reading

Boston Women's Health Book Collective, *The New Our Bodies Ourselves* (New York: Simon & Schuster, 1985)

Winnifred B. Cutler, Ph.D., *Hysterectomy: Before & After* (New York: Harper & Row, 1988)

Barbara Ehrenreich and Dierdre English, *For Her Own Good* (New York: Doubleday, 1979)

Charles Inlander et al., *Medicine on Trial* (Englewood Cliffs, N.J.: Prentice-Hall, 1988)

Herbert H. Keyser, M.D., *Women Under the Knife* (New York: Warner Books, 1986)

Susanne Morgan, Ph.D., *Coping with a Hysterectomy* (New York: New American Library, 1986)

Lynn Payer, *How to Avoid a Hysterectomy*, (New York: Pantheon, 1987)

Index